DIGITAL DETOX: RECLAIMING YOUR MIND AND BODY IN A HYPER-CONNECTED WORLD

INTRODUCTION: THE DIGITAL DILEMMA

Imagine waking up naturally with the sunrise, enjoying a leisurely breakfast without the constant buzz of notifications, and spending quality time with loved ones without the interruption of screens. For many, this idyllic scenario feels increasingly out of reach in our hyper-connected world.

In the past two decades, digital technology has revolutionized every aspect of our lives. From smartphones and social media to remote work and online education, our reliance on digital devices has become ubiquitous. While these advancements have brought undeniable benefits—enhancing communication, providing access to information, and fostering global connectivity—they have also introduced a host of challenges that impact our mental and physical well-being.

Digital addiction is a modern epidemic characterized by excessive and compulsive use of digital devices, leading to significant interference with daily life. Unlike substance addiction, digital addiction is often socially acceptable, making it harder to recognize and address. The constant barrage of notifications, the allure of endless scrolling, and the pressure to stay connected can create a cycle of dependency that is difficult to break.

Consider this: According to recent studies, the average person spends over four hours a day on their smartphone, a number that has steadily increased over the years. This excessive screen time is linked to a variety of health issues, including sleep disturbances, increased anxiety, and decreased attention spans. On a personal level, many of us have experienced the frustration of waking up to a flood of unread messages, the anxiety of being out of the loop, or the struggle to focus on tasks amidst constant digital interruptions.

The repercussions of digital overuse extend beyond individual health. Relationships can suffer as face-to-face interactions are replaced by virtual communication. Productivity declines when distractions become the norm, and creativity is stifled by the constant influx of information. Moreover, the quality of our leisure time diminishes when passive scrolling replaces meaningful activities like reading, exercising, or engaging in hobbies.

In a world where technology continues to advance at a rapid pace, the need to address digital overuse has never been more urgent. Ignoring the signs of digital addiction can lead to long-term consequences that affect every facet of our lives. By taking proactive steps to manage our digital consumption, we can reclaim control over our time, improve our mental and physical health, and foster deeper, more meaningful connections with others.

"Digital Detox: Reclaiming Your Mind and Body in a Hyper-Connected World" is designed to guide you through the process of reducing digital dependency and restoring balance in your life. This book offers actionable strategies, tailored detox plans, and mindfulness techniques to help you navigate the complexities of our digital landscape. Each chapter delves into different aspects of digital overuse, providing practical solutions to enhance your well-being and cultivate a healthier relationship with technology.

Embarking on a digital detox journey is not about rejecting technology but about finding harmony between our digital and real-life experiences. It's about making conscious choices that prioritize our health, relationships, and personal growth. As you turn the pages of this book, you'll discover the tools and insights needed to reclaim your mind and body, empowering you to live a more balanced and fulfilling life in our hyper-connected world.

CHAPTER 1: UNDERSTANDING DIGITAL OVERUSE

In today's fast-paced world, digital technology is seamlessly woven into the fabric of our daily lives. From the moment we wake up to the sound of our smartphones and the instant access to information and entertainment they provide, to the late-night scrolling that often disrupts our sleep, our interactions with digital devices are constant and pervasive. While these technologies offer numerous benefits, their overuse can lead to significant challenges that affect our mental, emotional, and physical well-being.

Defining Digital Addiction

Digital addiction, often referred to as internet addiction or screen addiction, is characterized by excessive and compulsive use of digital devices that interferes with daily life. Unlike traditional addictions, which are typically associated with substances like alcohol or drugs, digital addiction centers around behaviors such as excessive gaming, constant social media engagement, or relentless browsing. This form of addiction is insidious because it is socially accepted and even encouraged in many aspects of modern life, making it harder to recognize and address.

The scope of digital addiction is vast, encompassing various forms of technology use. It ranges from the overuse of smartphones and computers to the inability to disconnect from social media platforms and online communities. This addiction can manifest in different ways, including an overwhelming need to check notifications, a reluctance to engage in face-to-face interactions, and a persistent feeling of being tethered to the digital world.

Psychological Impacts of Digital Overuse

The psychological effects of digital overuse are profound and multifaceted. One of the most significant impacts is the increase in anxiety and stress levels. The constant barrage of information, notifications, and the pressure to stay connected can create a sense of overwhelm and urgency. This perpetual state of alertness can lead to heightened anxiety, making it difficult for individuals to relax and unwind.

Moreover, digital overuse can contribute to depression and feelings of loneliness. While social media platforms are designed to connect people, they can sometimes have the opposite effect. Superficial interactions and the comparison of one's life to the curated lives of others can lead to feelings of inadequacy and isolation. The lack of meaningful, face-to-face interactions can further exacerbate these feelings, creating a cycle of loneliness despite being constantly "connected."

Physiological Effects of Excessive Screen Time

Beyond the psychological ramifications, excessive screen time has tangible physiological effects. Prolonged use of digital devices can lead to poor posture, resulting in chronic back and neck pain. Eye strain and headaches are common issues caused by extended periods of looking at screens, particularly with inadequate lighting or improper screen settings.

Sleep disturbances are another critical consequence of digital overuse. The blue light emitted by screens interferes with the production of melatonin, the hormone responsible for regulating sleep. This disruption can lead to difficulties falling asleep, reduced sleep quality, and overall fatigue. The impact on sleep not only affects daily functioning but also contributes to longer-term health issues, including weakened immune systems and impaired cognitive function.

The Role of Social Media, Smartphones, and Other Digital Devices

Social media platforms, smartphones, and other digital devices play a central role in the phenomenon of digital overuse. Social media, in particular, is engineered to maximize user engagement through algorithms that promote endless scrolling and continuous interaction. Features like likes, shares, and notifications trigger the brain's reward system, making it difficult for users to disengage.

Smartphones serve as the gateway to this digital ecosystem, providing constant access to social media, games, news, and entertainment. The portability and multifunctionality of smartphones mean that digital engagement can occur anywhere and at any time, blurring the boundaries between work and personal life. This constant accessibility fosters habits of frequent checking and prolonged usage, contributing significantly to digital overuse.

Other digital devices, such as tablets, laptops, and gaming consoles, also contribute to the pervasive presence of technology in our lives. These devices facilitate not only work and education but also leisure and social interaction, making it challenging to establish healthy boundaries. The integration of technology into every aspect of life means that digital overuse can easily become ingrained in daily routines, making it harder to recognize and address.

Recognizing the Signs of Digital Overuse

Understanding digital overuse begins with recognizing its signs and symptoms. Common indicators include:

- **Constant Need to Check Devices:** Feeling compelled to check your phone or other devices frequently, even during inappropriate times like meetings or social gatherings.

- **Neglecting Responsibilities:** Allowing digital activities to interfere with work, studies, or personal responsibilities.

- **Sleep Disruptions:** Struggling to fall asleep or experiencing poor sleep quality due to late-night screen use.

- **Physical Discomfort:** Experiencing eye strain, headaches, or musculoskeletal issues from prolonged device use.

- **Emotional Distress:** Feeling anxious, stressed, or irritable when unable to access digital devices.

Recognizing these signs is the first step toward addressing digital overuse. It highlights the need for a conscious effort to create a healthier relationship with technology, which will be explored further in the subsequent chapters of this book.

The Path Forward

Understanding the depths of digital overuse is crucial for anyone seeking to reclaim their mind and body from the grips of a hyper-connected world. By acknowledging the definitions, psychological and physiological impacts, and the roles that various digital devices play, individuals can begin to identify the areas of their lives most affected by digital addiction. This awareness lays the foundation for developing effective strategies to reduce screen time, enhance real-life connections, and improve overall well-being.

In the chapters that follow, we will delve deeper into assessing personal digital habits, exploring the science behind digital detox, and implementing actionable plans to achieve a balanced and fulfilling life free from the constraints of digital overuse. The journey to reclaiming your mind and body starts with understanding the problem, and Chapter 1 serves as the essential first step in this transformative process.

CHAPTER 2: ASSESSING YOUR DIGITAL HABITS

Understanding your digital habits is the crucial first step in embarking on a successful digital detox journey. Before you can make meaningful changes, it's essential to gain a clear and honest picture of how you interact with digital devices and platforms daily. This chapter will guide you through the process of tracking your screen time, identifying patterns and triggers, and conducting self-assessment exercises to understand your unique relationship with technology.

The Importance of Self-Assessment

Before making any changes, it's vital to recognize how deeply integrated digital devices are in your life. Self-assessment allows you to:

- **Identify Usage Patterns:** Understand when, where, and how you use digital devices.

- **Recognize Triggers:** Pinpoint the situations or emotions that lead to increased screen time.

- **Measure Impact:** Assess how digital overuse affects

various aspects of your life, including productivity, relationships, and well-being.

- **Set Realistic Goals:** Establish achievable objectives based on your current habits and challenges.

Tools and Methods for Tracking Screen Time

To accurately assess your digital habits, you need reliable tools and methods to monitor your screen time. Here are some effective ways to track your digital usage:

1. Built-In Device Trackers

Most smartphones, tablets, and computers come with built-in tracking features that provide detailed insights into your screen time.

- **iOS (Screen Time):** Offers reports on app usage, notifications received, and device pickups. You can set limits for specific apps and categories.

- **Android (Digital Wellbeing):** Similar to iOS, it tracks app usage, notifications, and provides tools to set usage limits and focus modes.

- **Windows (Activity Report):** Windows 10 and later versions include features to monitor screen time and app usage.

- **macOS (Screen Time):** Provides insights into how much time you spend on each app and website.

2. Third-Party Applications

For more comprehensive tracking and additional features, consider using third-party apps:

- **RescueTime:** Runs in the background and tracks time spent on various applications and websites, providing detailed reports and productivity scores.

- **Moment:** Focuses on helping users reduce screen time by tracking usage and setting daily limits.

- **StayFree:** Offers detailed analytics on app usage and screen time, along with goal-setting features.

- **Forest:** Combines screen time tracking with a productivity tool that encourages you to stay off your phone by growing a virtual tree.

3. Manual Tracking

If you prefer a more hands-on approach, manual tracking can be effective:

- **Daily Logs:** Keep a journal where you note the time you spend on different digital activities throughout the day.

- **Time Blocking:** Allocate specific time blocks for digital usage and non-digital activities, then review your adherence to the schedule.

4. Browser Extensions

For those who spend significant time on their computers, browser extensions can help monitor and limit usage:

- **StayFocusd (Chrome):** Limits the amount of time you can spend on distracting websites.

- **LeechBlock (Firefox):** Blocks or restricts access to specified websites during set times.

- **TimeTracker (Various Browsers):** Tracks time spent on different websites and generates reports.

Identifying Patterns and Triggers

Once you've collected data on your digital habits, the next step is to analyze it to identify patterns and triggers that lead to excessive screen time.

1. Analyzing Usage Data

- **Peak Usage Times:** Determine the times of day when you are most active on digital devices. Are you using them more during mornings, afternoons, or evenings?

- **Popular Apps and Websites:** Identify which applications and websites consume the most of your time. Are there specific apps that you find hard to put down?

- **Device Dependency:** Assess which devices you rely on the most. Do you use your smartphone more than your computer or tablet?

2. Recognizing Emotional and Situational Triggers

Understanding the reasons behind your digital usage can help address the root causes of overuse.

- **Emotional Triggers:** Do you turn to digital devices when you're bored, stressed, lonely, or anxious? Identifying these emotions can help you find healthier coping mechanisms.

- **Situational Triggers:** Are there specific situations that lead to increased screen time, such as during meals, before bedtime, or while commuting?

- **Social Triggers:** Do notifications from social media or messaging apps prompt you to check your phone frequently?

3. Behavioral Patterns

Look for recurring behaviors that indicate a dependency on digital devices.

- **Automatic Checking:** Do you habitually check your phone for notifications without a specific reason?

- **Multitasking:** Do you often use multiple devices or switch between tasks, leading to fragmented attention?

- **Procrastination:** Do you use digital devices to avoid tasks or responsibilities?

Self-Assessment Exercises

Engage in self-assessment exercises to deepen your understanding of your digital habits and their impact on your life.

1. Digital Diary

Maintain a digital diary for at least one week where you record:

- **Duration:** How much time you spend on each digital device and application.

- **Activities:** The specific activities you engage in (e.g., social media, gaming, work-related tasks).

- **Emotions:** Your emotional state before, during, and after using digital devices.

- **Contexts:** The context in which you use digital devices (e.g., at home, during meals, while commuting).

Reviewing your diary at the end of the week can reveal patterns and areas where you can reduce or modify your usage.

2. Reflective Questions

Ask yourself the following questions to gain insight into your digital habits:

- **Purpose:** Why do I use digital devices? Is it for work, entertainment, social connection, or something else?

- **Necessity:** Is my digital usage necessary for my daily

tasks and responsibilities, or is it excessive?

- **Impact:** How does my screen time affect my mood, productivity, relationships, and physical health?
- **Control:** Do I feel in control of my digital usage, or does it control me?

3. Behavior Mapping

Create a behavior map to visualize the relationship between your digital habits and other aspects of your life.

- **Activities:** List all your daily activities and mark where digital device usage fits in.
- **Connections:** Draw connections between digital usage and outcomes like productivity, relaxation, social interactions, and health.
- **Patterns:** Identify any negative patterns where digital usage leads to undesirable outcomes.

4. Goal Setting

Based on your assessments, set specific, measurable, achievable, relevant, and time-bound (SMART) goals to modify your digital habits.

- **Example Goals:**
    - Reduce smartphone usage by 30 minutes each day within the next month.
    - Limit social media browsing to 15 minutes per session.
    - Implement a no-phone rule during meals and one hour before bedtime.

Assessing the Impact of Digital Overuse

To fully understand the need for a digital detox, assess how digital overuse currently affects different areas of your life.

1. Mental Health

- **Stress and Anxiety:** Increased screen time, especially on social media, can heighten feelings of stress and anxiety.

- **Attention Span:** Constant digital interruptions can reduce your ability to concentrate and maintain focus on tasks.

- **Mood Fluctuations:** Excessive use of digital devices can lead to mood swings and irritability, especially when unable to access them.

2. Physical Health

- **Sedentary Lifestyle:** Prolonged screen time often leads to a lack of physical activity, contributing to weight gain and related health issues.

- **Sleep Quality:** Blue light from screens can disrupt sleep patterns, leading to insufficient rest and fatigue.

- **Eye Strain and Posture:** Extended use of digital devices can cause eye strain, headaches, and poor posture, resulting in chronic pain.

3. Social Relationships

- **Isolation:** Paradoxically, increased digital interactions can lead to feelings of isolation and loneliness.

- **Communication Skills:** Overreliance on digital communication can hinder the development of effective interpersonal skills.

- **Quality Time:** Digital distractions can reduce the quality of time spent with family and friends, weakening relationships.

4. Productivity and Creativity

- **Distractions:** Frequent notifications and the temptation to multitask can disrupt workflow and decrease productivity.

- **Procrastination:** Digital devices can be a major source of procrastination, leading to unfinished tasks and missed deadlines.

- **Creative Blocks:** Constant exposure to information can overwhelm the brain, making it difficult to engage in creative thinking and problem-solving.

Creating a Baseline

Establishing a baseline of your current digital habits provides a reference point to measure your progress throughout the detox process.

1. Baseline Metrics

- **Total Screen Time:** Calculate your average daily screen time across all devices.

- **App Usage:** Identify the top apps and platforms that consume the most of your time.

- **Peak Usage Periods:** Note the times of day when your digital usage is highest.

2. Personal Reflection

Reflect on how your current digital habits align with your personal values and goals.

- **Alignment with Goals:** Are your digital habits helping or hindering your personal and professional goals?

- **Value Consistency:** Do your digital interactions reflect your core values and priorities?

3. Identifying Areas for Improvement

Based on your assessments, pinpoint specific areas where reducing digital usage can have the most significant positive impact.

- **High-Impact Changes:** Focus on changes that will yield substantial benefits, such as reducing social media time or eliminating unnecessary notifications.

- **Incremental Adjustments:** Start with small, manageable changes to avoid feeling overwhelmed.

Setting the Stage for Change

With a clear understanding of your digital habits and their impact, you're now prepared to begin making intentional changes. This chapter has equipped you with the tools and insights needed to assess your digital usage comprehensively. In the next chapter, we will explore the science behind digital detox, delving into how excessive digital use affects your brain and body, and the benefits of reducing screen time.

CHAPTER 3: THE SCIENCE OF DIGITAL DETOX

In our hyper-connected world, the integration of digital technology into every facet of our lives has profound implications for our brain and body. Understanding the science behind digital detox is essential to comprehend why reducing screen time is crucial for our overall well-being. This chapter delves into the physiological and neurological effects of excessive digital use, explores the myriad benefits of a digital detox, and examines the latest research findings that underscore the importance of reclaiming our lives from digital overuse.

How Excessive Digital Use Affects the Brain and Body

Excessive use of digital devices doesn't just occupy our time—it actively alters the very fabric of our brains and bodies. The constant interaction with screens and digital media can lead to a range of negative outcomes, both mentally and physically.

1. Neurological Impacts

a. Altered Brain Structure and Function

Prolonged screen time can lead to changes in brain structure and function. Studies have shown that excessive digital use, especially in children and adolescents, can affect areas of the brain responsible for attention, memory, and emotional regulation.

- **Reduced Attention Span:** Constant notifications and the habit of multitasking can impair the brain's ability to focus. The prefrontal cortex, which governs executive functions like decision-making and attention, can become less efficient with continuous digital distractions.

- **Impaired Memory:** Relying on digital devices for information storage can weaken the brain's natural memory processes. This phenomenon, often referred to as "digital amnesia," occurs when individuals are less likely to remember information they expect to find online.

b. Dopamine and Reward Systems

Digital interactions, particularly those involving social media, games, and other engaging content, trigger the brain's reward system by releasing dopamine—a neurotransmitter associated with pleasure and reinforcement.

- **Addictive Behaviors:** The intermittent rewards provided by likes, shares, and notifications can create addictive behaviors, encouraging users to seek constant digital engagement to achieve the same pleasurable feelings.

2. Psychological Impacts

a. Increased Anxiety and Stress

The perpetual connectivity enabled by digital devices can lead to heightened levels of anxiety and stress. The fear of missing out (FOMO) and the pressure to respond immediately to messages can create a constant state of alertness, preventing relaxation and increasing overall stress levels.

b. Depression and Loneliness

Paradoxically, while digital platforms aim to connect individuals, they can contribute to feelings of loneliness and depression. Superficial online interactions may replace meaningful face-to-face relationships, leading to a sense of isolation despite being constantly "connected."

3. Physical Health Consequences

a. Sleep Disruption

Exposure to blue light emitted by screens interferes with the production of melatonin, the hormone responsible for regulating sleep-wake cycles. This disruption can lead to difficulties falling asleep, reduced sleep quality, and insufficient rest.

b. Musculoskeletal Issues

Prolonged use of digital devices often results in poor posture, leading to chronic back, neck, and shoulder pain. Additionally, repetitive motions like typing or swiping can cause strain injuries such as carpal tunnel syndrome.

c. Eye Strain and Visual Problems

Extended screen time can cause digital eye strain, characterized by symptoms like dryness, irritation, blurred vision, and headaches. The constant focus on screens can also contribute to long-term visual problems, including myopia (nearsightedness).

Benefits of Reducing Screen Time

Embarking on a digital detox offers a multitude of benefits that enhance both mental and physical health. By consciously reducing screen time, individuals can experience significant improvements in various aspects of their lives.

1. Enhanced Cognitive Function

a. Improved Attention and Focus

Reducing digital distractions allows the brain to concentrate better on tasks, enhancing productivity and the ability to engage in deep work. This improved focus can lead to higher quality outcomes in both personal and professional endeavors.

b. Better Memory Retention

Engaging in activities that require active recall and critical thinking, rather than relying on digital storage, strengthens the brain's natural memory processes, leading to better information retention and cognitive resilience.

2. Emotional Well-Being

a. Decreased Anxiety and Stress

Less exposure to digital stimuli reduces the constant bombardment of information and the pressure to stay connected, leading to lower anxiety levels and enhanced emotional stability.

b. Increased Happiness and Life Satisfaction

Engaging in real-life activities, such as spending time with loved ones, pursuing hobbies, and being present in the moment, fosters a greater sense of fulfillment and happiness compared to passive digital consumption.

3. Physical Health Improvements

a. Better Sleep Quality

Reducing screen time, especially before bedtime, helps regulate sleep patterns, resulting in deeper, more restorative sleep and increased daytime energy levels.

b. Enhanced Physical Health

Less time spent sitting and staring at screens encourages more physical activity, which improves cardiovascular health, muscle strength, and overall fitness. Additionally, alleviating musculoskeletal strain contributes to long-term physical well-being.

4. Strengthened Relationships

a. Deeper Connections

Face-to-face interactions foster deeper, more meaningful relationships compared to digital communication. Building strong personal connections enhances emotional support and social fulfillment.

b. Improved Communication Skills

Engaging in in-person conversations enhances verbal and non-verbal communication skills, leading to more effective and empathetic interactions with others.

5. Increased Productivity and Creativity

a. Enhanced Productivity

With fewer digital distractions, individuals can allocate more time and mental resources to important tasks, leading to higher productivity and achievement of goals.

b. Boosted Creativity

Engaging in creative activities without the interruption of digital devices allows for more free-flowing and innovative thinking, fostering creativity and problem-solving abilities.

Research Findings on Digital Detox

Scientific research provides compelling evidence supporting the benefits of digital detox. Numerous studies have explored the effects of reducing screen time on various aspects of health and well-being.

1. Mental Health Studies

A study published in the *Journal of Behavioral Addictions* found that individuals who engaged in a digital detox reported significant reductions in anxiety and depression symptoms. The participants also experienced improvements in mood and overall life satisfaction.

2. Cognitive Function Research

Research conducted by the University of California demonstrated that limiting screen time enhances cognitive functions such as attention, memory, and executive control. Participants who reduced their digital usage showed marked improvements in task performance and information retention.

3. Sleep Quality Investigations

A study in the *Journal of Sleep Research* revealed that individuals who reduced screen time before bed experienced better sleep quality, including longer sleep duration and fewer sleep disturbances. The findings highlight the critical role of screen time management in maintaining healthy sleep patterns.

4. Physical Health Outcomes

The *American Journal of Preventive Medicine* published research indicating that decreased screen time is associated with increased physical activity levels, lower body mass index (BMI), and reduced risk of chronic diseases such as obesity and diabetes.

5. Social Interaction Studies

A study from the *American Journal of Psychiatry* found that reduced digital communication led to stronger interpersonal relationships and increased feelings of social support. Participants reported feeling more connected and less isolated when they prioritized in-person interactions over digital ones.

6. Longitudinal Studies

Long-term studies have shown that sustained digital detox practices contribute to lasting improvements in mental and physical health. Participants who maintained reduced screen time over several months continued to experience enhanced well-being and productivity.

The Neuroscience Behind Digital Detox

Understanding the neuroscience behind digital detox provides deeper insight into why reducing screen time is beneficial.

1. Neuroplasticity and Habit Formation

The brain's ability to reorganize itself by forming new neural connections—known as neuroplasticity—plays a crucial role in habit formation and change. By consciously reducing digital usage, individuals can rewire their brains to develop healthier habits and break the cycle of digital dependency.

2. Dopamine Regulation

Regular digital interactions can lead to dopamine dysregulation, where the brain becomes desensitized to dopamine rewards, requiring more frequent or intense stimuli to achieve the same pleasurable feelings. A digital detox helps restore dopamine balance, making everyday activities more rewarding and reducing the need for constant digital stimulation.

3. Stress Response System

Chronic digital overuse can hyperactivate the body's stress response system, leading to elevated cortisol levels and increased vulnerability to stress-related illnesses. Reducing screen time allows the stress response system to normalize, promoting better stress management and resilience.

4. Brain Connectivity and Functionality

Excessive screen time, especially involving multitasking, can impair the brain's connectivity and functionality. A digital detox enhances neural connectivity in areas responsible for focus, creativity, and emotional regulation, leading to improved cognitive and emotional health.

Implementing a Science-Based Digital Detox

Leveraging scientific insights can enhance the effectiveness of a digital detox. Here are evidence-based strategies to incorporate into your detox plan:

1. Gradual Reduction

Abruptly eliminating digital use can be overwhelming and unsustainable. Gradually reducing screen time allows the brain to adjust and develop new habits without significant stress.

2. Mindful Consumption

Be intentional about your digital use. Focus on consuming content that adds value to your life and minimizes time spent on passive or mindless browsing.

3. Scheduled Breaks

Incorporate regular digital-free periods into your daily routine. Scheduled breaks help prevent digital fatigue and promote mental rejuvenation.

4. Alternative Activities

Engage in activities that do not involve screens, such as reading, exercising, or pursuing hobbies. These activities stimulate different parts of the brain and contribute to overall well-being.

5. Digital Boundaries

Set clear boundaries for digital use, such as no devices during meals or one hour before bedtime. These boundaries help create a balanced relationship with technology.

6. Support Systems

Surround yourself with a supportive environment that encourages digital detox practices. Share your goals with friends and family to gain their support and accountability.

CHAPTER 4: CREATING A PERSONALIZED DETOX PLAN

Embarking on a digital detox journey requires more than just the desire to reduce screen time—it demands a structured and personalized approach. Creating a tailored detox plan ensures that the changes you implement are sustainable and effective in reclaiming your mind and body from digital overuse. This chapter will guide you through developing a step-by-step plan, setting realistic and achievable goals, and building a supportive environment to facilitate your digital detox.

The Importance of a Personalized Detox Plan

A one-size-fits-all approach rarely yields the best results, especially when it comes to changing deeply ingrained habits. A personalized detox plan takes into account your unique lifestyle, digital usage patterns, and personal goals. By customizing your approach, you increase the likelihood of success and make the process more manageable and less overwhelming.

- **Tailored Solutions:** Address your specific challenges and digital habits.

- **Increased Motivation:** Align your goals with your personal values and aspirations.

- **Sustainable Changes:** Implement strategies that fit seamlessly into your daily routine.

Step-by-Step Guide to Reducing Screen Time

Creating an effective detox plan involves several key steps. Follow this structured approach to systematically reduce your screen time and enhance your overall well-being.

1. Assess Your Current Digital Usage

Before making any changes, it's essential to understand your current digital habits. Refer back to Chapter 2, where you learned how to track and analyze your screen time.

- **Review Your Digital Diary:** Look for patterns in your usage data.

- **Identify High-Usage Areas:** Determine which apps or devices consume the most of your time.

- **Acknowledge Triggers:** Recognize the situations or emotions that lead to increased screen time.

2. Define Your Detox Goals

Setting clear and specific goals provides direction and motivation. Use the SMART criteria to ensure your goals are:

- **Specific:** Clearly define what you want to achieve.
  - *Example:* "I want to reduce my social media usage from 3 hours to 1 hour per day."

- **Measurable:** Ensure you can track your progress.
  - *Example:* "I will limit my smartphone screen time to 2 hours each day."

- **Achievable:** Set realistic goals that are attainable.

- *Example:* "I will replace 30 minutes of evening screen time with reading."

- **Relevant:** Align your goals with your personal values and needs.

  - *Example:* "Reducing screen time will help me spend more quality time with my family."

- **Time-Bound:** Set a deadline for achieving your goals.

  - *Example:* "I will achieve this reduction within the next four weeks."

3. Develop Actionable Strategies

Implementing effective strategies is crucial to reaching your detox goals. Here are some practical approaches:

a. Gradual Reduction

Instead of making drastic changes overnight, gradually decrease your screen time to make the transition smoother.

- **Week 1:** Reduce screen time by 15 minutes.

- **Week 2:** Decrease by an additional 15 minutes.

- **Week 3:** Cut down another 15 minutes.

- **Week 4:** Continue reducing until you reach your target screen time.

b. Implement Digital Boundaries

Establish clear boundaries to manage your digital usage effectively.

- **No-Device Zones:** Designate areas in your home where digital devices are not allowed, such as the dining room or bedroom.

- **Scheduled Downtime:** Allocate specific times of the

day when you disconnect from all digital devices, like during meals or one hour before bedtime.

- **Notification Management:** Turn off non-essential notifications to minimize distractions.

c. Utilize Technology to Your Advantage

Leverage apps and built-in device features to support your detox efforts.

- **Screen Time Apps:** Use tools like Screen Time (iOS) or Digital Wellbeing (Android) to monitor and limit your usage.

- **Focus Modes:** Enable features that block distracting apps during designated times.

- **Productivity Tools:** Apps like Forest or Freedom can help you stay focused by restricting access to certain websites or apps.

d. Replace Digital Activities with Meaningful Alternatives

Find fulfilling activities to substitute screen time, enhancing your overall well-being.

- **Physical Exercise:** Engage in regular physical activities like walking, yoga, or sports.

- **Hobbies:** Pursue interests such as reading, painting, gardening, or playing a musical instrument.

- **Social Interactions:** Spend quality time with friends and family through face-to-face interactions or phone calls instead of texting.

4. Create a Daily Routine

Establishing a consistent daily routine helps reinforce your detox plan and makes it easier to adhere to your goals.

- **Morning Routine:** Start your day without immediately reaching for your phone. Instead, engage in activities like stretching, meditation, or journaling.

- **Work/Study Schedule:** Allocate specific times for focused work and incorporate regular breaks to prevent digital fatigue.

- **Evening Wind-Down:** Develop a calming pre-sleep routine that excludes screen time, such as reading a book or practicing relaxation techniques.

5. Monitor and Adjust Your Plan

Regularly tracking your progress and making necessary adjustments ensures your detox plan remains effective.

- **Weekly Check-Ins:** Review your screen time data and assess your adherence to your goals.

- **Identify Challenges:** Recognize any obstacles or setbacks and develop strategies to overcome them.

- **Adjust Goals:** Modify your goals as needed to maintain motivation and ensure they remain achievable.

Setting Realistic Goals

Setting realistic and achievable goals is fundamental to the success of your digital detox. Unrealistic goals can lead to frustration and eventual abandonment of your detox efforts. Here's how to set goals that are both challenging and attainable:

1. Start Small

Begin with manageable changes that you can easily incorporate into your routine. Small successes build confidence and momentum for larger changes.

- **Example:** Reduce your daily social media use by 30 minutes instead of cutting it out entirely.

2. Prioritize Your Goals

Focus on the areas that have the most significant impact on your well-being. Identify which aspects of your digital usage are most detrimental and target them first.

- **Example:** If late-night screen time is affecting your sleep, prioritize reducing device usage before bedtime.

3. Be Flexible

Allow yourself the flexibility to adjust your goals based on your progress and any unforeseen challenges. Life is dynamic, and your detox plan should be adaptable.

- **Example:** If reducing screen time by 30 minutes is too challenging initially, start with a 15-minute reduction and gradually increase it.

4. Celebrate Milestones

Acknowledge and celebrate your achievements, no matter how small. Recognizing progress boosts motivation and reinforces positive behavior.

- **Example:** Treat yourself to a favorite activity or reward when you successfully reduce your screen time for a week.

5. Stay Accountable

Share your goals with a trusted friend or family member who can support and hold you accountable. Accountability partners can provide encouragement and help you stay on track.

- **Example:** Check in with your accountability partner weekly to discuss your progress and any challenges you're facing.

Building a Support System

A strong support system plays a crucial role in the success of your digital detox. Surrounding yourself with individuals who understand and support your goals can provide the encouragement and accountability needed to stay committed.

1. Involve Friends and Family

Communicate your detox goals to those around you and enlist their support.

- **Explain Your Goals:** Share why you're embarking on a digital detox and how they can support you.

- **Set Boundaries Together:** Encourage your loved ones to join you in reducing screen time, creating a shared commitment to digital wellness.

2. Join Support Groups

Connecting with others who are also pursuing a digital detox can provide motivation and a sense of community.

- **Online Communities:** Participate in forums, Facebook groups, or Discord servers dedicated to digital detox and wellness.

- **Local Groups:** Attend local meetups or workshops focused on reducing screen time and promoting digital balance.

3. Seek Professional Help if Needed

If you find it particularly challenging to reduce digital usage, consider seeking help from a mental health professional.

- **Therapists and Counselors:** Professionals can provide strategies and support to address underlying issues related to digital addiction.

- **Coaches and Mentors:** Digital wellness coaches can offer personalized guidance and accountability.

4. Leverage Technology for Support

Use apps and tools that promote accountability and provide

support throughout your detox journey.

- **Accountability Apps:** Apps like Habitica or StickK allow you to set goals and receive reminders to stay on track.

- **Supportive Features:** Enable features on your devices that encourage digital wellness, such as bedtime modes or focus sessions.

Creating a Sustainable Detox Plan

A successful digital detox isn't a temporary fix but a long-term lifestyle change. Here are strategies to ensure your detox plan is sustainable:

1. Integrate Detox Practices into Daily Life

Incorporate digital detox strategies into your daily routine so they become habitual.

- **Consistent Scheduling:** Maintain regular digital-free periods each day.

- **Routine Adjustments:** Adapt your routine as needed to accommodate changes in your lifestyle or schedule.

2. Reflect and Adapt

Regular reflection helps you understand what's working and what isn't, allowing you to make necessary adjustments.

- **Journaling:** Keep a journal to document your experiences, challenges, and successes.

- **Feedback Loops:** Seek feedback from your support system to gain different perspectives on your progress.

3. Maintain Flexibility

Life can be unpredictable, and flexibility is key to maintaining your detox plan amidst changes.

- **Adjust Goals:** Modify your goals based on your current situation and progress.

- **Be Kind to Yourself:** Acknowledge that setbacks are part of the journey and don't let them derail your efforts.

4. Focus on Overall Well-Being

A digital detox should enhance your overall well-being, not just reduce screen time. Focus on holistic wellness practices that support your mental, emotional, and physical health.

- **Balanced Lifestyle:** Incorporate a mix of activities that promote balance, such as exercise, hobbies, social interactions, and relaxation techniques.

- **Mindfulness Practices:** Engage in mindfulness and meditation to stay present and reduce the urge to engage in digital activities mindlessly.

5. Set Long-Term Goals

Beyond your initial detox plan, set long-term goals to maintain a balanced digital lifestyle.

- **Ongoing Assessment:** Periodically review your digital habits and make adjustments as needed.

- **Continuous Improvement:** Strive for continuous improvement in your relationship with technology, seeking ways to enhance your digital wellness.

CHAPTER 5: MINDFULNESS AND DIGITAL MINIMALISM

In the quest to reclaim your mind and body from the grips of digital overuse, mindfulness and digital minimalism emerge as powerful allies. These practices offer structured approaches to cultivate awareness, intentionality, and simplicity in your interactions with technology. This chapter explores the principles of mindfulness and digital minimalism, providing you with practical techniques and strategies to integrate these concepts into your daily life, thereby fostering a balanced and fulfilling digital lifestyle.

Understanding Mindfulness

Mindfulness is the practice of being fully present and engaged in the current moment, aware of your thoughts, feelings, and sensations without judgment. It involves cultivating a heightened state of awareness that allows you to respond to situations with clarity and intention rather than reacting impulsively.

Benefits of Mindfulness in Digital Detox

- **Enhanced Self-Awareness:** Recognize your digital habits and the triggers that lead to overuse.

- **Improved Focus:** Increase your ability to concentrate on tasks without constant digital interruptions.

- **Emotional Regulation:** Manage stress, anxiety, and other emotions that may drive excessive screen time.

- **Greater Presence:** Foster deeper connections with yourself and others by being fully engaged in real-life interactions.

Principles of Digital Minimalism

Digital minimalism is a philosophy that advocates for the intentional use of technology to support your values and goals while minimizing distractions and unnecessary digital clutter. It emphasizes quality over quantity in your digital interactions, promoting a more meaningful and purposeful relationship with technology.

Core Principles of Digital Minimalism

1. **Intentionality:** Use digital tools purposefully, aligning their use with your personal values and objectives.

2. **Selective Engagement:** Choose to engage with only those digital platforms and activities that add significant value to your life.

3. **Simplification:** Reduce digital clutter by decluttering your digital spaces, such as organizing apps, unsubscribing from unnecessary notifications, and streamlining your online presence.

4. **Boundaries:** Establish clear boundaries for digital usage to create a balanced separation between your digital and real-life activities.

Integrating Mindfulness into Digital Usage

Mindfulness can transform how you interact with digital devices, making your usage more intentional and less habitual. Here are several mindfulness techniques to help you achieve a healthier digital balance:

1. Mindful Consumption

Approach digital content with intention rather than passively consuming it. Before opening an app or browsing the internet, pause and ask yourself:

- **Purpose:** Why am I using this digital tool right now?

- **Benefit:** What do I hope to gain from this activity?

- **Value:** Does this usage align with my personal values and goals?

By asking these questions, you can make conscious decisions about your digital consumption, ensuring that it serves a meaningful purpose.

2. Digital Mindfulness Breaks

Incorporate regular mindfulness breaks into your day to reduce digital fatigue and enhance mental clarity.

- **Breathing Exercises:** Take a few minutes to focus on your breath, inhaling deeply and exhaling slowly.

- **Body Scans:** Perform a quick scan of your body to identify and release tension.

- **Grounding Techniques:** Engage your senses by noticing what you can see, hear, feel, smell, and taste in your immediate environment.

These breaks help you reconnect with the present moment and diminish the urge to constantly check your devices.

3. Mindful Device Usage

Transform your interaction with digital devices by being fully present during their use.

- **Single-Tasking:** Focus on one digital task at a time instead of multitasking, which can lead to decreased productivity and increased stress.

- **Purposeful Engagement:** Use devices for specific tasks rather than aimlessly browsing or scrolling.

- **Conscious Pauses:** Before responding to a notification or message, take a moment to consider if and how you want to engage.

4. Digital Sabbaticals

Periodically disconnect from digital devices to reset your relationship with technology.

- **Short-Term Breaks:** Take a few hours each day to go device-free, allowing your mind to rest from constant digital stimulation.

- **Extended Retreats:** Plan longer digital detoxes, such as weekends or vacations, where you significantly reduce or eliminate digital usage.

Digital sabbaticals provide an opportunity to experience life without the constant presence of digital distractions, fostering a deeper sense of well-being and presence.

Embracing Digital Minimalism

Adopting digital minimalism involves making intentional choices about the technologies you use and how you use them. Here are practical strategies to implement digital minimalism in your life:

1. Audit Your Digital Life

Conduct a thorough audit of your digital devices, applications, and online activities to identify areas where you can simplify and declutter.

- **Device Assessment:** Evaluate which devices you genuinely need and use regularly.

- **App Evaluation:** Review all installed applications and remove those that do not add significant value.

- **Subscription Review:** Cancel subscriptions to services and newsletters that no longer serve your interests or needs.

2. Streamline Your Digital Spaces

Create organized and efficient digital environments to reduce clutter and enhance productivity.

- **Organize Apps and Files:** Categorize and arrange your apps and digital files in a way that makes them easy to access and use.

- **Simplify Interfaces:** Customize your device interfaces to highlight essential tools and minimize distractions.

- **Manage Notifications:** Turn off non-essential notifications to prevent constant interruptions and maintain focus.

3. Prioritize Quality over Quantity

Focus on engaging with high-quality digital content that enriches your life rather than accumulating a vast amount of low-value interactions.

- **Curate Your Feed:** Follow accounts and channels that inspire, educate, or entertain you meaningfully.

- **Limit Media Consumption:** Set boundaries on the amount of time you spend consuming digital media, ensuring it aligns with your personal goals and interests.

- **Engage Purposefully:** Participate in digital activities that foster genuine connections and personal growth.

4. Establish Digital Boundaries

Set clear and consistent boundaries to create a balanced relationship with technology.

- **Designated Device-Free Times:** Allocate specific times of the day when digital devices are not allowed, such as during meals or before bedtime.

- **No-Device Zones:** Create physical spaces in your home where digital devices are prohibited, promoting face-to-face interactions and relaxation.

- **Work-Life Balance:** Separate work-related digital activities from personal time to prevent burnout and maintain mental well-being.

5. Foster Real-Life Connections

Prioritize real-life interactions over digital communication to build deeper and more meaningful relationships.

- **Face-to-Face Meetings:** Choose in-person meetings or phone calls over text messages or social media interactions whenever possible.

- **Quality Time with Loved Ones:** Dedicate uninterrupted time to spend with family and friends, enhancing emotional bonds and support systems.

- **Community Engagement:** Participate in local

events, clubs, or volunteer opportunities to strengthen your sense of community and belonging.

Mindfulness Practices to Support Digital Minimalism

Integrating mindfulness practices can reinforce your commitment to digital minimalism by fostering a greater sense of awareness and intentionality.

1. Meditation

Regular meditation practice enhances focus, reduces stress, and promotes a calm and centered mind.

- **Daily Meditation:** Allocate time each day for meditation sessions, focusing on breath, sensations, or guided visualizations.

- **Mindful Breathing:** Incorporate mindful breathing exercises throughout the day to regain focus and reduce digital cravings.

2. Journaling

Journaling helps you reflect on your digital habits, track progress, and explore your emotions related to technology use.

- **Daily Reflections:** Write about your digital interactions, noting what worked well and what challenges you faced.

- **Goal Setting:** Use journaling to set and review your digital minimalism goals, celebrating achievements and identifying areas for improvement.

3. Gratitude Practice

Cultivating gratitude shifts your focus from digital distractions to appreciating the present moment and the positive aspects of your life.

- **Gratitude Journals:** List things you are grateful for each day, emphasizing real-life experiences and relationships.

- **Expressing Gratitude:** Share your appreciation with others, fostering stronger connections and reducing reliance on digital validation.

Case Studies and Real-Life Examples

To illustrate the transformative power of mindfulness and digital minimalism, consider the following case studies:

Case Study 1: Sarah's Journey to Mindful Tech Use

Sarah, a 35-year-old marketing professional, found herself constantly tethered to her smartphone, struggling to disconnect even during family time. By incorporating mindfulness techniques such as mindful consumption and scheduled digital breaks, Sarah was able to reduce her screen time by 50%. She noticed significant improvements in her relationships, sleep quality, and overall stress levels. Her mindful approach allowed her to use technology more intentionally, aligning her digital habits with her personal values.

Case Study 2: John's Adoption of Digital Minimalism

John, a college student, was overwhelmed by the sheer number of apps and notifications on his devices, leading to decreased productivity and increased anxiety. He decided to adopt digital minimalism by conducting a comprehensive audit of his digital life. John streamlined his apps, turned off unnecessary notifications, and established digital boundaries such as no-device zones during study sessions. These changes resulted in enhanced focus, better academic performance, and a more balanced lifestyle.

Implementing Mindfulness and Digital Minimalism: Actionable Steps

To help you integrate mindfulness and digital minimalism into your digital detox journey, here are practical steps to follow:

1. Start with Self-Awareness

- **Mindful Observation:** Pay attention to your digital habits without judgment. Notice how often you check your devices and what prompts you to do so.

- **Identify Patterns:** Recognize recurring patterns and triggers that lead to excessive digital use.

2. Set Intentional Goals

- **Define Your Why:** Understand why you want to practice mindfulness and digital minimalism. Whether it's to reduce stress, improve relationships, or enhance productivity, having a clear purpose will guide your efforts.

- **Create Specific Goals:** Set clear and measurable goals, such as reducing social media time by 30 minutes daily or implementing device-free evenings.

3. Develop Mindful Practices

- **Incorporate Meditation:** Allocate time each day for meditation to cultivate mindfulness and reduce digital cravings.

- **Practice Mindful Consumption:** Before using a digital device, pause and consider your intention and the value it brings to your life.

4. Simplify Your Digital Environment

- **Declutter Your Devices:** Remove unnecessary apps, organize your home screen, and streamline your digital tools.

- **Manage Notifications:** Turn off non-essential notifications to minimize distractions and regain control over your attention.

5. Establish Boundaries

- **Designate Digital-Free Times and Zones:** Create specific times and spaces where digital devices are not allowed, promoting real-life interactions and relaxation.

- **Set Usage Limits:** Use built-in device features or third-party apps to set daily limits on screen time and app usage.

6. Replace Digital Habits with Meaningful Activities

- **Engage in Hobbies:** Pursue interests that do not involve screens, such as reading, gardening, or exercising.

- **Foster Real-Life Connections:** Spend quality time with friends and family through face-to-face interactions or phone calls.

7. Monitor Progress and Reflect

- **Track Your Habits:** Use journals or digital trackers to monitor your progress and identify areas for improvement.

- **Reflect Regularly:** Assess how mindfulness and digital minimalism are impacting your well-being and make necessary adjustments.

8. Seek Support

- **Join Communities:** Connect with others who are also practicing mindfulness and digital minimalism for mutual support and accountability.

- **Share Your Journey:** Communicate your goals and progress with friends and family to garner their support and encouragement.

Overcoming Challenges in Practicing Mindfulness and Digital

Minimalism

Implementing mindfulness and digital minimalism can present several challenges. Here are strategies to overcome common obstacles:

1. Dealing with Resistance

- **Acknowledge Resistance:** Recognize that resistance is a natural part of change. Understand the reasons behind your reluctance to reduce digital use.

- **Stay Committed:** Remind yourself of your goals and the benefits of practicing mindfulness and digital minimalism to stay motivated.

2. Managing Urges and Cravings

- **Delay Response:** When you feel the urge to check your device, delay for a few minutes. This pause can help reduce impulsive behavior.

- **Engage in an Alternative Activity:** Replace the urge with a non-digital activity, such as taking a walk or practicing deep breathing.

3. Coping with Social Pressures

- **Communicate Your Goals:** Let others know about your digital detox efforts to garner their understanding and support.

- **Find Like-Minded Individuals:** Surround yourself with people who share your commitment to digital wellness.

4. Maintaining Consistency

- **Create Routines:** Incorporate mindfulness and digital minimalism practices into your daily routine to build consistency.

- **Be Patient:** Understand that forming new habits

takes time. Celebrate small victories and remain patient with yourself.

The Synergy of Mindfulness and Digital Minimalism

Mindfulness and digital minimalism complement each other, creating a synergistic effect that enhances your ability to manage digital overuse effectively. Mindfulness fosters awareness and intentionality, while digital minimalism provides a structured framework for simplifying and optimizing your digital interactions. Together, they empower you to create a harmonious balance between technology and real-life experiences, leading to improved mental and physical well-being.

Conclusion: Embracing a Mindful and Minimalist Digital Lifestyle

Integrating mindfulness and digital minimalism into your life is a transformative journey that requires dedication, self-awareness, and intentionality. By practicing mindfulness, you cultivate a deeper understanding of your digital habits and the motivations behind them. Embracing digital minimalism allows you to simplify your digital environment, prioritize meaningful interactions, and reduce unnecessary distractions. Together, these practices empower you to reclaim control over your digital usage, fostering a balanced and fulfilling lifestyle free from the constraints of digital overuse.

As you continue your digital detox journey, remember that mindfulness and digital minimalism are not destinations but ongoing practices that evolve with your changing needs and circumstances. Stay committed to your goals, remain adaptable, and celebrate the positive changes you achieve along the way. By doing so, you pave the way for a healthier, more intentional, and enriched life in our hyper-connected world.

CHAPTER 6: IMPROVING SLEEP THROUGH DIGITAL REDUCTION

Sleep is a fundamental pillar of health, essential for cognitive function, emotional well-being, and physical restoration. In our hyper-connected world, digital devices have become ubiquitous companions, often intruding into the most sacred hours of rest. This chapter explores the profound impact of digital overuse on sleep quality and provides actionable strategies to enhance your sleep hygiene by reducing screen time. By implementing these techniques, you can reclaim restful nights and wake up refreshed, ready to embrace each day with vitality.

The Impact of Screens on Sleep Quality

The advent of smartphones, tablets, and other digital devices has revolutionized the way we live, work, and communicate. However, this technological integration comes at a cost—our sleep quality. Understanding how digital devices interfere with sleep is crucial for anyone seeking to improve their overall well-being.

1. Blue Light and Melatonin Suppression

a. What is Blue Light?

Blue light is a high-energy visible (HEV) light emitted by digital screens, including smartphones, tablets, computers, and televisions. While blue light plays a role in regulating our circadian rhythms—our internal biological clocks—it can also disrupt these rhythms when exposure occurs at inappropriate times.

b. Melatonin Production

Melatonin is a hormone produced by the pineal gland in the brain, responsible for regulating sleep-wake cycles. Exposure to blue light in the evening suppresses melatonin production, making it harder to fall asleep and reducing sleep quality.

c. Research Findings

Studies have demonstrated that individuals exposed to blue light before bedtime experience delayed sleep onset, reduced sleep duration, and poorer sleep quality. For example, a study published in the *Journal of Applied Physiology* found that participants who used blue light-emitting devices for two hours before bedtime had significantly lower melatonin levels and took longer to fall asleep compared to those who engaged in non-screen activities.

2. Mental Stimulation and Sleep Onset

Engaging with digital content, whether through social media, gaming, or work-related tasks, stimulates the brain, making it more challenging to wind down. The mental alertness induced by interactive activities can delay the transition from wakefulness to sleep, leading to difficulties in falling asleep and fragmented sleep patterns.

3. Emotional Engagement and Stress

Digital interactions can evoke strong emotional responses, from excitement and joy to stress and anxiety. Engaging with emotionally charged content before bed can increase cortisol levels—the stress hormone—hindering relaxation and making it harder to achieve restful sleep.

Techniques for Better Sleep Hygiene

Improving sleep hygiene involves adopting habits and practices that promote consistent, uninterrupted, and restorative sleep. By reducing digital device usage before bedtime, you can significantly enhance your sleep quality. Here are several evidence-based strategies to achieve better sleep hygiene:

1. Establish a Digital Curfew

a. Define Screen-Free Hours

Set a specific time each evening to stop using digital devices, ideally at least one hour before bedtime. This period allows your body to begin winding down without the interference of blue light and mental stimulation.

b. Gradual Reduction

If abruptly eliminating screen time before bed is challenging, start by reducing usage gradually. For example, decrease your screen time by 15 minutes each week until you reach your desired digital curfew.

2. Use Blue Light Filters

a. Software Solutions

Many devices offer built-in blue light filtering options, such as Night Shift on iOS, Night Light on Windows, and Night Mode on Android. These settings reduce blue light emission by shifting the screen's color temperature to warmer tones.

b. Third-Party Applications

Consider using third-party apps like f.lux or Twilight, which automatically adjust your screen's color temperature based on the time of day, further minimizing blue light exposure.

3. Create a Bedtime Routine

a. Consistent Sleep Schedule

Maintain a consistent sleep schedule by going to bed and waking up at the same times each day, even on weekends. This regularity reinforces your body's natural circadian rhythms.

b. Relaxing Activities

Incorporate relaxing activities into your bedtime routine to signal to your body that it's time to wind down. Examples include:

- **Reading a Book:** Choose a physical book or an e-reader with low blue light emission.

- **Meditation:** Practice mindfulness or guided meditation to calm the mind.

- **Gentle Stretching:** Engage in light stretching or yoga to release physical tension.

4. Optimize Your Sleep Environment

a. Dark, Quiet, and Cool

Ensure your bedroom is conducive to sleep by keeping it dark, quiet, and cool. Use blackout curtains, earplugs, or white noise machines if necessary.

b. Comfortable Bedding

Invest in a comfortable mattress and pillows that support restful sleep. The quality of your bedding can significantly impact your sleep comfort and duration.

5. Limit Caffeine and Heavy Meals Before Bed

a. Avoid Stimulants

Limit the intake of caffeine and other stimulants in the hours leading up to bedtime, as they can interfere with your ability to fall asleep.

b. Light Snacks

If you're hungry before bed, opt for a light snack that promotes sleep, such as a banana, a small bowl of oatmeal, or a glass of warm milk.

6. Engage in Physical Activity

Regular physical activity during the day can promote better sleep at night. However, avoid vigorous exercise close to bedtime, as it can increase adrenaline levels and make it harder to fall asleep.

7. Manage Stress and Anxiety

Incorporate stress-management techniques into your daily routine to reduce anxiety and promote relaxation. Practices such as journaling, deep breathing exercises, and progressive muscle relaxation can be beneficial.

Creating a Bedtime Routine Without Digital Devices

Developing a structured bedtime routine that excludes digital devices can enhance your ability to fall asleep faster and enjoy deeper, more restorative sleep. Here's how to create an effective digital-free bedtime routine:

1. Wind Down with Non-Screen Activities

Choose activities that promote relaxation and disconnect you from digital stimulation:

- **Reading:** Select a physical book, magazine, or use an e-reader with minimal blue light.

- **Listening to Music:** Play calming music or nature sounds to create a serene atmosphere.

- **Engaging in Hobbies:** Spend time on hobbies like knitting, drawing, or puzzles that do not involve screens.

2. Practice Mindfulness and Relaxation Techniques

Incorporate mindfulness practices into your bedtime routine to ease the transition to sleep:

- **Meditation:** Allocate 10-15 minutes for guided meditation or silent reflection.

- **Breathing Exercises:** Practice deep breathing techniques to calm your nervous system.

- **Progressive Muscle Relaxation:** Sequentially tense and relax different muscle groups to release physical tension.

3. Set Up a Technology-Free Zone

Designate your bedroom as a technology-free zone to prevent digital intrusion during sleep hours:

- **Remove Devices:** Keep smartphones, tablets, and laptops out of the bedroom.

- **Alternative Charging Station:** Charge your devices in another room to reduce temptation.

- **Use Traditional Alarm Clocks:** Replace your smartphone alarm with a traditional alarm clock to avoid unnecessary screen exposure in the morning.

4. Create a Visual Cue for Sleep Time

Use visual cues to signal the end of your day and the beginning of your sleep routine:

- **Dim the Lights:** Lower the brightness of your room lights an hour before bedtime to mimic natural sunset and promote melatonin production.

- **Candles or Essential Oils:** Use scented candles or essential oils like lavender to create a calming environment.

5. Establish Consistent Pre-Sleep Habits

Develop consistent habits that prepare your body and mind for sleep:

- **Hydration:** Drink a glass of water to stay hydrated but avoid excessive fluids that may disrupt sleep.

- **Personal Hygiene:** Engage in a nightly hygiene routine, such as brushing your teeth and washing your face, to reinforce the transition to sleep.

Research Findings on Digital Reduction and Sleep Improvement

Scientific research underscores the critical relationship between digital device usage and sleep quality. Here are some key studies that highlight the benefits of reducing screen time for better sleep:

1. Blue Light and Sleep Study

A study published in the *Journal of Clinical Endocrinology & Metabolism* found that exposure to blue light in the evening significantly suppressed melatonin production and delayed sleep onset in participants. Those who used blue light-blocking glasses experienced improved sleep duration and quality compared to the control group.

2. Digital Curfew Research

Research conducted by the University of Toledo demonstrated that implementing a digital curfew—turning off electronic devices one hour before bedtime—resulted in participants falling asleep faster, experiencing deeper sleep, and feeling more rested upon waking.

3. Sleep Hygiene Interventions

A meta-analysis published in the *Sleep Medicine Reviews* reviewed multiple studies on sleep hygiene interventions, concluding that reducing screen time before bed is consistently associated with better sleep outcomes, including increased sleep duration and reduced sleep latency.

4. Longitudinal Sleep Studies

Long-term studies have shown that sustained reduction in digital device usage before bedtime leads to lasting improvements in sleep quality. Participants who maintained reduced screen time over several months continued to experience enhanced sleep patterns and overall well-being.

Implementing a Science-Based Sleep Improvement Plan

Leveraging scientific insights can enhance the effectiveness of your sleep improvement efforts. Here are evidence-based strategies to incorporate into your plan:

1. Gradual Adjustment of Screen Time

Rather than making abrupt changes, gradually reduce your screen time before bed to allow your body to adjust:

- **Week 1:** Limit device usage to one hour before bedtime.

- **Week 2:** Decrease to 45 minutes before bed.

- **Week 3:** Further reduce to 30 minutes before bed.

- **Week 4:** Aim for 15 minutes before bed or implement a complete digital curfew.

2. Optimize Lighting

Adjust the lighting in your environment to support natural sleep cues:

- **Warm Lighting:** Use lamps with warm-colored bulbs in the evening to minimize blue light exposure.

- **Dimmer Switches:** Install dimmer switches to control the brightness levels in your home as the day progresses.

3. Incorporate Physical Relaxation Techniques

Engage in activities that promote physical relaxation and prepare your body for sleep:

- **Stretching:** Perform gentle stretches to relieve muscle tension.

- **Yoga:** Practice restorative yoga poses that enhance relaxation.

4. Monitor Sleep Patterns

Track your sleep patterns to identify improvements and areas for further adjustment:

- **Sleep Journals:** Maintain a sleep journal to record bedtime, wake time, sleep quality, and any factors affecting your sleep.

- **Sleep Tracking Devices:** Use wearable devices or smartphone apps to monitor sleep duration and quality.

5. Seek Professional Guidance if Needed

If sleep issues persist despite implementing digital reduction strategies, consider seeking help from a sleep specialist or healthcare professional:

- **Cognitive Behavioral Therapy for Insomnia (CBT-I):** A structured program that helps individuals identify and change thoughts and behaviors that affect their sleep.

- **Medical Evaluation:** Rule out underlying health conditions that may be contributing to sleep disturbances.

CHAPTER 7: ENHANCING REAL-LIFE CONNECTIONS

In an era dominated by digital interactions, the quality and depth of our real-life connections have been significantly impacted. While technology has made it easier to stay in touch with people across the globe, it has also led to a paradoxical sense of isolation and superficial relationships. Enhancing real-life connections is essential for emotional well-being, personal growth, and overall happiness. This chapter explores the importance of face-to-face interactions, the detrimental effects of digital overuse on relationships, and provides actionable strategies to cultivate and strengthen meaningful real-life connections.

The Importance of Real-Life Connections

Human beings are inherently social creatures, thriving on meaningful interactions and relationships. Real-life connections offer a depth and authenticity that digital interactions often lack. They provide emotional support, foster a sense of belonging, and contribute to mental and physical health.

1. Emotional Support and Well-Being

- **Deep Emotional Bonds:** Face-to-face interactions allow for the expression of genuine emotions, fostering deeper emotional bonds and trust between individuals.

- **Mental Health Benefits:** Strong real-life connections are linked to lower rates of anxiety, depression, and stress. They provide a support system that can help individuals navigate life's challenges.

- **Physical Health Improvements:** Engaging in meaningful relationships can lead to better immune function, reduced blood pressure, and increased longevity.

2. Sense of Belonging and Community

- **Community Engagement:** Participating in community activities and building local connections enhances your sense of belonging and purpose.

- **Identity and Self-Esteem:** Real-life interactions contribute to a stronger sense of identity and higher self-esteem, as individuals receive validation and affirmation from others.

3. Personal Growth and Development

- **Skill Building:** Interacting with others in person helps develop essential social skills, such as empathy, active listening, and effective communication.

- **Diverse Perspectives:** Engaging with a diverse range of people broadens your understanding of the world, fostering open-mindedness and adaptability.

The Effects of Digital Overuse on Relationships

While digital technology offers convenience, excessive use can undermine the quality of our relationships and social interactions.

1. Superficial Interactions

- **Lack of Depth:** Digital conversations often lack the emotional depth and non-verbal cues present in face-to-face interactions, leading to more superficial relationships.

- **Quantity Over Quality:** The focus on maintaining numerous online connections can detract from nurturing a few deep and meaningful relationships.

2. Reduced Presence and Attention

- **Distraction:** Constant digital distractions, such as checking smartphones during conversations, diminish the quality of interactions and signal a lack of interest.

- **Attention Fragmentation:** Multitasking with digital devices during social interactions can lead to fragmented attention and reduced engagement.

3. Miscommunication and Misunderstandings

- **Lack of Non-Verbal Cues:** Digital communication often lacks non-verbal cues like body language and facial expressions, increasing the likelihood of misunderstandings.

- **Delayed Responses:** Asynchronous communication can lead to delayed responses and misinterpretations of intent and tone.

4. Increased Isolation Despite Connectivity

- **Paradox of Choice:** The abundance of online connections can create a false sense of social fulfillment, leading individuals to neglect in-person relationships.

- **Loneliness:** Relying heavily on digital interactions can result in feelings of loneliness and social isolation, even when surrounded by online connections.

Strategies to Enhance Real-Life Connections

Rebuilding and strengthening real-life connections requires intentional effort and the implementation of specific strategies to prioritize face-to-face interactions.

1. Prioritize Face-to-Face Interactions

- **Schedule Regular Meetups:** Set aside dedicated time each week to meet friends and family in person.

- **Limit Digital Communication:** Reduce the frequency of online interactions and focus on in-person conversations.

2. Create Opportunities for Social Engagement

- **Join Clubs and Groups:** Participate in clubs, hobby groups, or community organizations that align with your interests.

- **Attend Social Events:** Make an effort to attend social gatherings, such as parties, networking events, and community festivals.

3. Improve Communication Skills

- **Active Listening:** Practice active listening by fully concentrating on the speaker, understanding their message, and responding thoughtfully.

- **Express Empathy:** Show empathy by acknowledging others' feelings and perspectives, fostering deeper emotional connections.

4. Foster Meaningful Conversations

- **Ask Open-Ended Questions:** Encourage deeper discussions by asking questions that require more than yes or no answers.

- **Share Personal Stories:** Open up about your experiences and encourage others to do the same, building trust and intimacy.

5. Be Present During Interactions

- **Limit Multitasking:** Focus solely on the person you are interacting with, avoiding distractions like checking your phone.

- **Mindful Presence:** Practice mindfulness during conversations to stay engaged and fully present in the moment.

6. Strengthen Existing Relationships

- **Quality Time:** Spend quality time with loved ones by engaging in shared activities that promote bonding.

- **Show Appreciation:** Regularly express gratitude and appreciation for the people in your life to reinforce positive connections.

7. Build New Relationships

- **Step Out of Your Comfort Zone:** Take the initiative to meet new people by attending events, volunteering, or taking up new hobbies.

- **Be Approachable:** Cultivate an open and friendly demeanor to make it easier for others to connect with you.

Practical Steps to Foster Meaningful Interactions

Implementing practical steps can facilitate the enhancement of real-life connections and ensure sustained improvement in your social relationships.

1. Set Relationship Goals

- **Define What You Want:** Determine the type of relationships you want to cultivate, such as deep friendships, supportive family bonds, or professional networks.

- **Create Action Plans:** Develop specific actions to achieve these goals, such as reaching out to a friend once a week or attending networking events monthly.

2. Allocate Time for Social Activities

- **Daily Interactions:** Incorporate short, meaningful interactions into your daily routine, such as having a meal with family without digital distractions.

- **Weekly Commitments:** Commit to regular social activities, such as a weekly coffee date with a friend or a monthly game night.

3. Engage in Shared Activities

- **Collaborative Projects:** Work on projects or activities that require teamwork, fostering collaboration and camaraderie.

- **Group Hobbies:** Participate in group hobbies, such as sports, book clubs, or art classes, to build connections around shared interests.

4. Practice Gratitude in Relationships

- **Express Thanks:** Regularly thank people for their support, presence, and contributions to your life.

- **Acknowledge Milestones:** Celebrate important milestones and achievements with your loved ones to strengthen bonds.

5. Develop Empathetic Relationships

- **Understand Perspectives:** Make an effort to understand and respect others' viewpoints and experiences.

- **Offer Support:** Be there for others during challenging times, offering emotional support and practical assistance.

Overcoming Challenges in Enhancing Real-Life Connections

Strengthening real-life connections can present several challenges, especially in a digital-centric society. Here are strategies to overcome common obstacles:

1. Time Constraints

- **Prioritize Relationships:** Recognize the importance of relationships and make them a priority in your schedule.

- **Efficient Time Management:** Use effective time management techniques to balance social interactions with other responsibilities.

2. Social Anxiety and Shyness

- **Gradual Exposure:** Slowly increase your participation in social settings to build confidence.

- **Seek Support:** Consider seeking support from a therapist or joining a social skills group to overcome anxiety.

3. Maintaining Consistency

- **Set Reminders:** Use calendars or reminders to ensure you consistently engage in social activities.

- **Accountability Partners:** Partner with a friend to

hold each other accountable for maintaining social commitments.

4. Balancing Digital and Real-Life Interactions

- **Digital Boundaries:** Establish clear boundaries for digital usage to prevent it from encroaching on real-life interactions.

- **Intentional Use:** Use digital tools intentionally to support, rather than replace, real-life connections.

Case Studies and Real-Life Examples

To illustrate the transformative power of enhancing real-life connections, consider the following case studies:

Case Study 1: Emily's Journey to Reconnect

Emily, a 28-year-old graphic designer, found herself feeling isolated despite having numerous online friends. Realizing the superficiality of her digital interactions, she decided to prioritize real-life connections. Emily joined a local art class and started attending weekly meetups. Through these activities, she developed meaningful friendships, experienced increased happiness, and felt more connected to her community.

Case Study 2: Michael's Strengthened Family Bonds

Michael, a 45-year-old manager, noticed that his family's interactions were becoming increasingly dominated by digital devices. Determined to improve his family's relationships, he implemented a "no-device dinner" rule and organized monthly family outings. These changes led to deeper conversations, stronger emotional bonds, and a more harmonious family dynamic.

Implementing Strategies to Enhance Real-Life Connections: Actionable Steps

To help you integrate the strategies discussed into your life, here are practical steps to follow:

1. Assess Your Current Relationships

- **Evaluate Relationship Quality:** Reflect on the quality and depth of your existing relationships.

- **Identify Gaps:** Determine which relationships need strengthening and which new connections you wish to cultivate.

2. Set Clear Relationship Goals

- **Define Objectives:** Clearly outline what you want to achieve in your relationships, such as deeper connections or expanded social circles.

- **Create a Plan:** Develop a step-by-step plan to reach these goals, including specific actions and timelines.

3. Take Initiative in Social Settings

- **Initiate Conversations:** Don't wait for others to reach out—take the first step in starting conversations and making plans.

- **Be Open and Approachable:** Cultivate a friendly demeanor to make it easier for others to connect with you.

4. Allocate Dedicated Time for Relationships

- **Schedule Social Time:** Block out specific times in your calendar dedicated to social interactions.

- **Be Present:** During social activities, focus on being fully present and engaged with others.

5. Practice Active Listening and Empathy

- **Listen Fully:** Give your full attention to the speaker without interrupting or planning your response.

- **Show Understanding:** Acknowledge and validate others' feelings and perspectives to foster trust and intimacy.

6. Engage in Shared Experiences

- **Plan Activities:** Organize activities that you and others enjoy, creating opportunities for bonding and shared memories.

- **Collaborate on Projects:** Work together on projects or goals that require teamwork and cooperation.

7. Maintain and Nurture Relationships

- **Regular Check-Ins:** Reach out regularly to friends and family to maintain connections.

- **Celebrate Successes:** Acknowledge and celebrate the achievements and milestones of those you care about.

Conclusion: The Power of Real-Life Connections

Enhancing real-life connections is a vital component of a successful digital detox journey. By prioritizing face-to-face interactions, fostering meaningful relationships, and implementing intentional strategies, you can rebuild and strengthen the bonds that contribute to your emotional and physical well-being. Real-life connections provide the support, fulfillment, and sense of belonging that digital interactions alone cannot offer. As you continue your journey to reclaim your mind and body from digital overuse, remember that investing in your real-life relationships is investing in your overall happiness and health.

CHAPTER 8: BOOSTING OVERALL WELL-BEING

Reclaiming your mind and body from digital overuse is not just about reducing screen time—it's about enhancing your overall well-being. Digital detox serves as a gateway to a healthier, more balanced lifestyle that nurtures your mental, emotional, and physical health. This chapter explores how digital reduction can significantly boost your well-being, highlighting the interconnectedness of various health dimensions and providing actionable strategies to cultivate a fulfilling and harmonious life.

Understanding Overall Well-Being

Overall well-being is a multifaceted concept that encompasses various dimensions of health. Achieving balance across these dimensions leads to a flourishing life where you experience positive emotions, a sense of purpose, healthy relationships, and engagement in meaningful activities.

1. The Holistic Nature of Well-Being

- **Mental Health:** Involves cognitive functions,

emotional stability, and psychological resilience.

- **Emotional Health:** Pertains to managing emotions, maintaining positive relationships, and experiencing fulfillment.

- **Physical Health:** Relates to bodily well-being, including exercise, nutrition, and sleep.

- **Social Health:** Concerns the quality of relationships and social interactions.

- **Spiritual Health:** Involves a sense of purpose, values, and connection to something greater.

By addressing digital overuse, you can create space for practices and habits that promote holistic health, leading to a synergistic improvement in all aspects of your life.

2. The Impact of Digital Overuse on Well-Being

Excessive digital usage can disrupt the balance across these well-being dimensions, leading to a decline in overall health and happiness.

- **Mental Health Decline:** Increased anxiety, depression, and cognitive fatigue.

- **Emotional Instability:** Heightened stress levels and reduced emotional resilience.

- **Physical Health Issues:** Sedentary lifestyle, poor posture, and disrupted sleep patterns.

- **Social Isolation:** Superficial relationships and decreased face-to-face interactions.

- **Reduced Productivity:** Frequent distractions and impaired focus leading to decreased efficiency.

Addressing digital overuse is a critical step toward reversing these negative impacts and fostering a healthier, more balanced life.

Mental Health Improvements

Reducing digital dependency can lead to significant enhancements in mental health, promoting a clearer, more focused mind and reducing the prevalence of mental health issues.

1. Decreased Anxiety and Depression

Excessive screen time, particularly on social media, is linked to increased feelings of anxiety and depression. Constant exposure to curated content can lead to comparisons, feelings of inadequacy, and a fear of missing out (FOMO). By limiting digital interactions, you reduce these stressors and create a more stable emotional environment.

- **Research Insight:** A study published in the *Journal of Social and Clinical Psychology* found that reducing social media usage led to significant decreases in both anxiety and depression symptoms.

2. Enhanced Cognitive Function

Frequent digital distractions can impair cognitive functions such as attention, memory, and problem-solving skills. Minimizing digital interruptions allows your brain to engage in deeper, more meaningful thought processes.

- **Improved Focus:** With fewer digital distractions, your ability to concentrate on tasks improves, leading to higher productivity and better quality work.

- **Better Memory Retention:** Engaging in activities that require active recall and critical thinking enhances your memory and cognitive resilience.

3. Increased Emotional Resilience

Digital detox fosters emotional resilience by allowing you to process emotions more effectively without the constant input of digital stimuli. This leads to better stress management and a more balanced emotional state.

- **Mindfulness Practices:** Incorporating mindfulness techniques during a digital detox can further enhance emotional regulation and resilience.

Physical Health Improvements

Digital overuse often leads to a sedentary lifestyle and various physical health issues. Reducing screen time can pave the way for healthier habits and improved physical well-being.

1. Increased Physical Activity

Less time spent on screens means more time available for physical activities, which are essential for maintaining a healthy body.

- **Exercise Benefits:** Regular physical activity improves cardiovascular health, strengthens muscles, and enhances flexibility.

- **Weight Management:** Engaging in exercise helps in maintaining a healthy weight and reducing the risk of obesity-related diseases.

2. Better Posture and Reduced Pain

Prolonged use of digital devices can lead to poor posture, resulting in chronic back, neck, and shoulder pain. By limiting device usage, you can reduce the strain on your body and adopt healthier posture habits.

- **Ergonomic Practices:** Incorporating ergonomic setups and regular breaks can further alleviate physical discomfort.

3. Enhanced Sleep Quality

Digital detox significantly improves sleep quality by reducing exposure to blue light and mental stimulation before bedtime.

- **Restorative Sleep:** Better sleep leads to improved immune function, increased energy levels, and overall physical restoration.

Emotional Well-Being

Emotional well-being is closely tied to your relationships and personal fulfillment. Reducing digital overuse can lead to a more balanced emotional state and deeper connections with others.

1. Greater Life Satisfaction

Engaging in meaningful, real-life activities enhances your sense of purpose and fulfillment, leading to greater overall life satisfaction.

- **Engagement in Hobbies:** Pursuing interests and hobbies that do not involve screens fosters a sense of accomplishment and joy.

2. Improved Mood Regulation

Less digital exposure reduces the fluctuations in mood caused by overuse of technology, leading to a more stable and positive emotional state.

- **Stress Reduction:** Engaging in relaxing, non-digital activities helps in lowering stress levels and promoting a calm mind.

Social Health Enhancements

Building and maintaining meaningful real-life connections is vital for social health. Digital detox allows you to nurture these relationships more effectively.

1. Stronger Relationships

Face-to-face interactions foster deeper emotional bonds and trust, enhancing the quality of your relationships.

- **Quality Time:** Spending uninterrupted time with loved ones strengthens connections and fosters mutual support.

2. Enhanced Communication Skills

Real-life interactions improve your verbal and non-verbal communication skills, leading to more effective and empathetic interactions.

- **Active Listening:** Practicing active listening during conversations enhances understanding and reduces misunderstandings.

Productivity and Creativity Boosts

Reducing digital distractions can lead to significant improvements in productivity and creativity, allowing you to achieve more and think more creatively.

1. Increased Productivity

With fewer interruptions, you can focus more intently on tasks, leading to higher efficiency and better work outcomes.

- **Deep Work:** Engaging in periods of uninterrupted work enhances your ability to perform complex tasks and achieve higher-quality results.

2. Enhanced Creativity

A clear, focused mind fosters creativity, allowing you to think outside the box and develop innovative solutions.

- **Creative Practices:** Engaging in creative activities such as writing, painting, or brainstorming sessions stimulates creative thinking.

Long-Term Benefits and Sustaining Well-Being

The benefits of a digital detox extend beyond immediate improvements, contributing to long-term health and well-being. Sustaining these benefits requires ongoing commitment and the integration of healthy habits into your daily life.

1. Establishing Healthy Digital Habits

Developing and maintaining healthy digital habits ensures that the positive changes achieved during a detox are sustained over time.

- **Consistent Boundaries:** Maintaining clear boundaries for digital usage helps prevent relapse into excessive screen time.

- **Regular Assessments:** Periodically evaluating your digital habits allows you to make necessary adjustments and stay on track.

2. Continuing Personal Growth

A digital detox opens up opportunities for continuous personal growth and self-improvement, fostering a lifelong commitment to well-being.

- **Lifelong Learning:** Engaging in continuous learning and self-development activities enhances personal fulfillment and growth.

- **Adaptability:** Cultivating adaptability and resilience helps you navigate the ever-evolving digital landscape without compromising your well-being.

3. Building a Supportive Environment

Creating a supportive environment that encourages healthy habits and well-being is essential for maintaining the benefits of a digital detox.

- **Community Support:** Surrounding yourself with like-minded individuals provides encouragement and accountability.

- **Positive Reinforcement:** Celebrating your

achievements and milestones reinforces positive behavior and motivates continued progress.

Case Studies and Real-Life Examples

To illustrate the transformative power of digital detox in boosting overall well-being, consider the following case studies:

Case Study 1: Lisa's Path to Enhanced Well-Being

Lisa, a 32-year-old teacher, struggled with high stress levels and poor sleep quality due to constant digital engagement. By implementing a digital detox plan, she reduced her screen time by 50%, established a consistent bedtime routine, and engaged in regular physical activities. As a result, Lisa experienced reduced anxiety, improved sleep quality, increased energy levels, and stronger relationships with her family and friends.

Case Study 2: David's Journey to Greater Productivity and Creativity

David, a 40-year-old software developer, found his productivity declining due to frequent digital distractions. He decided to limit his use of social media and implement scheduled digital-free periods during work hours. This led to a significant increase in his productivity, allowing him to complete projects more efficiently. Additionally, David noticed a boost in his creativity, enabling him to develop innovative solutions and ideas in his work.

Case Study 3: Maria's Transformation Through Holistic Wellness

Maria, a 27-year-old graphic designer, felt overwhelmed by the demands of her digital-centric job, leading to burnout and diminished creativity. She embarked on a digital detox journey, incorporating mindfulness practices, physical exercise, and real-life social interactions into her daily routine. Over time, Maria regained her creative spark, experienced improved mental clarity, and cultivated a balanced lifestyle that enhanced both her personal and professional life.

Implementing Strategies to Boost Overall Well-Being:

Actionable Steps

To help you integrate the strategies discussed into your life, here are practical steps to follow:

1. Conduct a Well-Being Assessment

- **Evaluate Your Current State:** Reflect on your well-being across various dimensions—mental, emotional, physical, social, and spiritual.

- **Identify Areas for Improvement:** Determine which aspects of your well-being need the most attention and prioritize them in your detox plan.

2. Set Comprehensive Well-Being Goals

- **Holistic Objectives:** Define goals that address multiple dimensions of well-being, such as improving mental health, enhancing physical fitness, and fostering meaningful relationships.

- **SMART Goals:** Ensure your goals are Specific, Measurable, Achievable, Relevant, and Time-bound to facilitate effective progress tracking.

3. Develop a Balanced Routine

- **Incorporate Diverse Activities:** Create a daily routine that includes a mix of work, physical activity, hobbies, social interactions, and relaxation.

- **Allocate Time Wisely:** Ensure that each activity has designated time slots, balancing digital and non-digital engagements.

4. Practice Mindfulness and Self-Care

- **Regular Mindfulness Practices:** Engage in daily mindfulness exercises such as meditation, deep breathing, or yoga to enhance self-awareness and emotional regulation.

- **Self-Care Rituals:** Prioritize self-care activities that rejuvenate your mind and body, such as taking baths, reading, or enjoying nature.

5. Foster Meaningful Relationships

- **Invest in Connections:** Dedicate time and effort to build and maintain strong relationships with family, friends, and community members.

- **Engage Authentically:** Interact with others authentically, showing genuine interest and empathy to deepen your connections.

6. Enhance Physical Health

- **Regular Exercise:** Incorporate physical activities into your routine, such as walking, running, cycling, or participating in fitness classes.

- **Healthy Nutrition:** Maintain a balanced diet that supports your physical and mental health, avoiding excessive caffeine and sugar.

7. Prioritize Sleep and Rest

- **Consistent Sleep Schedule:** Maintain a regular sleep schedule by going to bed and waking up at the same times each day.

- **Create a Restful Environment:** Ensure your sleeping environment is comfortable, dark, quiet, and cool to promote restful sleep.

8. Limit Digital Exposure

- **Set Digital Boundaries:** Establish clear boundaries for digital device usage, such as no screens during meals or one hour before bedtime.

- **Use Technology Mindfully:** Be intentional about your digital consumption, focusing on activities that add value and minimizing passive scrolling or mindless browsing.

9. Engage in Continuous Learning and Growth

- **Pursue New Skills:** Engage in activities that promote learning and personal growth, such as taking up a new hobby, attending workshops, or enrolling in online courses.

- **Reflect and Adapt:** Regularly assess your progress and make adjustments to your well-being plan as needed to stay aligned with your goals.

10. Build a Supportive Network

- **Seek Support:** Surround yourself with individuals who support your well-being goals and encourage your progress.

- **Join Communities:** Participate in groups or communities focused on well-being, digital detox, or personal development to gain additional support and resources.

Overcoming Challenges in Boosting Well-Being

Enhancing overall well-being through digital detox can present several challenges. Here are strategies to overcome common obstacles:

1. Dealing with Resistance to Change

- **Understand the Benefits:** Remind yourself of the positive outcomes that boosting your well-being can bring to your life.

- **Start Small:** Begin with manageable changes to build confidence and momentum.

2. Maintaining Consistency

- **Set Reminders:** Use alarms or notifications to

remind yourself to adhere to your well-being routines.

- **Create Habits:** Incorporate well-being activities into your daily routine until they become habitual.

3. Managing Time Effectively

- **Prioritize Tasks:** Focus on high-priority tasks that align with your well-being goals.

- **Use Time Management Tools:** Utilize planners, calendars, or apps to organize your schedule and allocate time for well-being activities.

4. Coping with Setbacks

- **Stay Resilient:** Accept that setbacks are part of the journey and use them as learning opportunities.

- **Seek Support:** Reach out to your support network for encouragement and assistance during challenging times.

5. Balancing Digital and Non-Digital Activities

- **Intentional Scheduling:** Allocate specific times for digital activities and ensure ample time for non-digital engagements.

- **Mindful Transitions:** Transition mindfully between digital and non-digital activities to maintain balance and focus.

The Synergy of Digital Detox and Overall Well-Being

Digital detox and overall well-being are intrinsically linked, with each enhancing the other in a synergistic manner. By reducing digital overuse, you create the necessary space and mental clarity to focus on activities and habits that promote holistic health. In turn, improved well-being reinforces your commitment to maintaining a balanced digital lifestyle, creating a positive feedback loop that sustains your progress.

Conclusion: Embracing a Life of Enhanced Well-Being

Boosting overall well-being through digital detox is a transformative endeavor that touches every aspect of your life. By addressing mental, emotional, physical, and social health, you create a foundation for a fulfilling and balanced existence. The strategies and insights provided in this chapter empower you to take intentional steps toward enhancing your well-being, fostering a harmonious relationship with technology, and embracing a life rich in health, happiness, and personal growth.

As you continue your digital detox journey, remember that the pursuit of well-being is ongoing. Stay committed to your goals, remain adaptable to change, and continuously seek opportunities for personal development. By doing so, you not only reclaim your mind and body from digital overuse but also cultivate a life of sustained well-being and fulfillment.

CHAPTER 9: OVERCOMING CHALLENGES AND RELAPSE

Embarking on a digital detox journey is a commendable step toward reclaiming your mind and body from the grips of digital overuse. However, like any significant lifestyle change, it comes with its own set of challenges and potential setbacks. This chapter delves into the common obstacles you might encounter during your digital detox, explores the reasons behind relapses, and provides effective strategies to overcome these hurdles. By understanding and addressing these challenges, you can maintain your commitment and achieve lasting success in your journey toward a balanced digital lifestyle.

Understanding the Nature of Challenges and Relapse

Change, especially when it involves altering deeply ingrained habits, is rarely smooth. Challenges and occasional setbacks are natural parts of the transformation process. Recognizing that these hurdles are temporary and manageable can empower you to navigate them with resilience and determination.

1. Common Challenges in Digital Detox

Several obstacles can impede your progress during a digital detox. Understanding these challenges can help you prepare and develop strategies to address them effectively.

- **Habitual Patterns:** Long-standing habits of checking devices frequently can be hard to break.

- **Social Pressure:** Friends, family, and colleagues may unintentionally encourage excessive digital use.

- **Work Demands:** Professional responsibilities often require constant connectivity, making it difficult to limit screen time.

- **Emotional Triggers:** Stress, boredom, or loneliness can drive you to seek comfort in digital interactions.

- **Accessibility and Convenience:** The omnipresence of digital devices makes it easy to revert to old habits, especially in environments where technology is readily available.

2. The Psychology Behind Relapse

Relapse is a common phenomenon in behavior change processes. Understanding the psychological factors that contribute to relapse can help you develop strategies to prevent it.

- **Cognitive Dissonance:** Holding conflicting thoughts about your digital habits can lead to inconsistency in your efforts.

- **Lack of Immediate Rewards:** The benefits of digital detox, such as improved well-being, are often long-term, making it challenging to stay motivated.

- **All-or-Nothing Thinking:** Believing that any lapse

means total failure can discourage continued efforts after a minor setback.

- **Emotional Coping Mechanism:** Using digital devices to manage negative emotions can reinforce dependency, making relapse more likely during stressful times.

Strategies to Overcome Challenges and Prevent Relapse

Successfully navigating challenges and preventing relapse requires a proactive approach, self-compassion, and the implementation of effective strategies. Here are comprehensive techniques to help you stay on track.

1. Develop a Strong Mindset

Cultivating a resilient and positive mindset is crucial for overcoming challenges and avoiding relapse.

- **Embrace a Growth Mindset:** View challenges as opportunities for growth rather than insurmountable obstacles. This perspective fosters resilience and adaptability.

*"Every setback is a setup for a comeback."

- **Stay Patient and Persistent:** Understand that change takes time. Celebrate small victories and remain committed, even when progress seems slow.

*"Consistency is more important than perfection."

- **Practice Self-Compassion:** Be kind to yourself during setbacks. Acknowledge your efforts and treat yourself with the same understanding you would offer a friend.

*"It's okay to stumble; what matters is that you get back up."

2. Implement Practical Strategies

Adopting specific strategies can help you manage challenges and reduce the likelihood of relapse.

a. Set Clear Boundaries

Establishing clear boundaries around digital usage can create a structured environment conducive to your detox goals.

- **Designate Tech-Free Zones:** Create spaces in your home where digital devices are not allowed, such as the dining room or bedroom.

Example: Transform your bedroom into a sanctuary by removing smartphones and tablets, encouraging restful sleep and undisturbed relaxation.

- **Define Tech-Free Times:** Allocate specific periods during the day when you disconnect from all digital devices, such as during meals or one hour before bedtime.

Example: Implement a "no screens during dinner" rule to foster meaningful conversations and strengthen family bonds.

- **Use Physical Barriers:** Keep devices out of immediate reach to reduce the temptation to check them frequently.

Example: Place your phone in another room while working or engaging in hobbies to maintain focus.

b. Create a Supportive Environment

Surrounding yourself with a supportive network can provide encouragement and accountability.

- **Communicate Your Goals:** Share your detox plans with friends and family to gain their understanding and support.

Example: Let your close friends know about your digital detox journey so they can respect your boundaries and support your efforts.

- **Find an Accountability Partner:** Partner with someone who shares similar goals to monitor each other's progress and offer mutual support.

Example: Pair up with a friend to check in weekly about your digital usage and celebrate each other's successes.

- **Join Support Groups:** Participate in online or local groups focused on digital detox and wellness to connect with like-minded individuals.

Example: Join a local wellness group or an online forum dedicated to digital detox to share experiences and gain insights.

c. Develop Healthy Coping Mechanisms

Replacing digital interactions with healthier alternatives can help you manage emotional triggers without reverting to old habits.

- **Engage in Physical Activity:** Exercise releases endorphins, which can improve your mood and reduce the urge to seek digital comfort.

Example: Start a daily walk or yoga routine to boost your physical and mental well-being.

- **Practice Mindfulness and Meditation:** These practices enhance self-awareness and emotional regulation, helping you respond to stress more effectively.

Example: Incorporate a 10-minute morning meditation to center yourself and set a positive tone for the day.

- **Pursue Hobbies:** Investing time in activities you enjoy can provide fulfillment and reduce reliance on digital devices for entertainment.

Example: Take up painting, gardening, or playing a musical instrument to engage your creativity and relax your mind.

d. Manage Work and Professional Responsibilities

Balancing digital detox with work demands is essential for sustained success.

- **Set Work Boundaries:** Define specific times for work-related digital usage and avoid extending it beyond those periods.

Example: Establish a rule to check work emails only during designated hours, preventing work from encroaching on personal time.

- **Utilize Productivity Tools:** Use tools like task managers and focus apps to enhance productivity without increasing digital consumption.

Example: Implement the Pomodoro Technique using a timer to break work into focused intervals with short breaks.

- **Communicate with Employers:** Inform your employer about your detox goals and negotiate flexible work arrangements if necessary.

Example: Discuss setting clear boundaries for after-hours communication to ensure you have time to unwind.

3. Develop Relapse Prevention Plans

Even with the best strategies, relapse can occur. Having a plan in place can help you recover quickly and get back on track.

- **Identify Warning Signs:** Recognize the early signs of potential relapse, such as increased stress or frequent device checking.

Example: Notice if you're feeling more anxious or starting to check your phone more often than usual.

- **Have a Recovery Plan:** Outline specific steps to take if you find yourself slipping back into old habits, such as taking a short break or reaching out to a support person.

Example: If you catch yourself scrolling mindlessly, pause, take deep breaths, and engage in a physical activity instead.

- **Learn from Setbacks:** Analyze what led to the relapse and adjust your strategies accordingly to prevent future occurrences.

Example: Reflect on a setback to understand triggers and develop targeted strategies to address them.

4. Foster Long-Term Commitment

Maintaining a digital detox is an ongoing process that requires sustained commitment and adaptability.

- **Regularly Reevaluate Goals:** Periodically assess your detox goals to ensure they align with your evolving needs and circumstances.

Example: Every few months, review your digital usage patterns and adjust your goals to continue improving.

- **Stay Informed:** Keep abreast of the latest research and strategies related to digital wellness to enhance your approach.

Example: Read books, attend workshops, or follow experts on digital wellness to stay motivated and informed.

- **Celebrate Progress:** Acknowledge and celebrate your achievements, no matter how small, to reinforce your commitment and motivation.

Example: Reward yourself with a favorite activity or treat when you successfully maintain your screen time limits for a week.

Case Studies and Real-Life Examples

To illustrate the effectiveness of these strategies, consider the following case studies:

Case Study 1: Emma's Battle with Social Media Addiction

Emma, a 25-year-old marketing professional, found herself spending upwards of five hours daily on social media platforms. This excessive use led to decreased productivity, anxiety, and strained relationships. Determined to regain control, Emma implemented a digital detox plan that included setting daily time limits, turning off non-essential notifications, and engaging in offline hobbies like painting and hiking. Despite initial challenges and a few relapses, Emma's consistent efforts led to a significant reduction in screen time, improved mental health, and stronger personal connections.

"I realized that my constant scrolling was draining me more than it was fulfilling. Setting limits and finding joy in offline activities transformed my daily life." – Emma

Case Study 2: Tom's Struggle with Work-Related Screen Time

Tom, a 40-year-old software engineer, struggled to disconnect from work-related digital tasks, even during off-hours. This constant connectivity resulted in burnout and poor sleep quality. Tom decided to establish clear work boundaries by setting a strict end time for work-related activities and designating weekends as digital-free periods. He also sought support from his employer to implement flexible work hours. While Tom faced difficulties adjusting initially, the structured approach helped him reduce burnout symptoms, improve sleep, and enhance his overall well-being.

"Setting boundaries was challenging, but it was essential for my mental and physical health. Now, I feel more balanced and energized." – Tom

Case Study 3: Sarah's Emotional Dependency on Digital Devices

Sarah, a 30-year-old graphic designer, used her smartphone as a primary coping mechanism for stress and loneliness. This dependency led to compulsive checking and interrupted her daily routines. Sarah sought professional help and joined a support group focused on digital wellness. She incorporated mindfulness practices and physical activities into her daily life, which helped her manage emotions without relying on digital devices. Over time, Sarah developed healthier coping mechanisms, reduced her screen time, and experienced improved emotional stability.

"I realized I was using my phone to numb my feelings. Finding healthier ways to cope made a huge difference in my emotional well-being." – Sarah

Implementing Strategies to Overcome Challenges: Actionable Steps

To help you integrate the strategies discussed into your life, here are practical steps to follow:

1. Conduct a Self-Assessment

- **Evaluate Your Digital Habits:** Reflect on your current digital usage patterns, identifying areas of overuse and triggers that lead to excessive screen time.

  Exercise: Complete the "Digital Habits Self-Assessment" worksheet (see Appendix A) to gain insight into your usage patterns.

- **Identify Personal Challenges:** Determine the specific challenges you face in your digital detox journey, such as habitual device checking or work-related digital demands.

Reflection Prompt: What are the top three challenges you face in reducing your digital usage?

2. Set Realistic and Flexible Goals

- **Define Clear Objectives:** Establish specific, measurable goals that address your unique challenges, such as reducing social media usage by one hour daily or implementing device-free zones in your home.

Example Goal: "I will reduce my social media usage from 3 hours to 1 hour per day over the next four weeks."

- **Allow Flexibility:** Recognize that setbacks are part of the process and adjust your goals as needed to accommodate your progress and changing circumstances.

Tip: If reducing screen time by an hour feels overwhelming, start with a 30-minute reduction and gradually increase it.

3. Develop a Comprehensive Support System

- **Communicate with Loved Ones:** Share your detox goals with friends and family to gain their understanding and support.

Example: Inform your family about your "no phones during dinner" rule to foster a supportive environment.

- **Find an Accountability Partner:** Partner with someone who shares similar goals to monitor each other's progress and offer mutual support.

Exercise: Create a weekly check-in schedule with your accountability partner to discuss progress and challenges.

- **Join Support Groups:** Engage with communities focused on digital detox to connect with like-minded individuals and gain additional support.

Resource: Consider joining online forums like the Digital Wellness Collective or local wellness meetups.

4. Create a Structured Plan

- **Establish Boundaries:** Define specific times and spaces where digital devices are limited or prohibited.

Example: Designate your living room as a tech-free zone to encourage in-person interactions.

- **Implement Practical Strategies:** Use techniques such as setting screen time limits, turning off non-essential notifications, and replacing digital activities with offline alternatives.

Tip: Use apps like "Forest" to stay focused by growing a virtual tree when you avoid using your phone.

- **Schedule Regular Check-Ins:** Set aside time each week to review your progress, identify challenges, and adjust your strategies accordingly.

Exercise: Use a weekly planner to track your screen time and reflect on your progress every Sunday evening.

5. Practice Mindfulness and Self-Compassion

- **Engage in Mindfulness Practices:** Incorporate activities like meditation, deep breathing, or yoga to enhance self-awareness and emotional regulation.

Exercise: Start a daily 5-minute meditation practice using guided apps like Headspace or Calm.

- **Be Kind to Yourself:** Acknowledge your efforts and

treat yourself with understanding and compassion, especially during setbacks.

Reflection Prompt: How can you show kindness to yourself when facing a setback in your digital detox journey?

6. Monitor Your Progress

- **Track Your Screen Time:** Use built-in device trackers or third-party apps to monitor your digital usage and assess your progress toward your goals.

Resource: Utilize apps like "Moment" or "RescueTime" to gain detailed insights into your screen time habits.

- **Reflect on Your Experiences:** Maintain a journal to document your journey, noting successes, challenges, and insights gained along the way.

Exercise: Start a "Digital Detox Journal" to record your daily digital usage, feelings, and reflections.

7. Adapt and Evolve

- **Stay Flexible:** Be willing to adjust your strategies based on what works best for you and your evolving needs.

Tip: If a particular strategy isn't working, experiment with alternative approaches until you find what suits you best.

- **Seek Continuous Improvement:** Continuously explore new techniques and strategies to enhance your digital detox efforts and overall well-being.

Resource: Read books like "Digital Minimalism" by Cal Newport or "The Power of Habit" by Charles Duhigg for further insights.

8. Seek Professional Support

- **Consult a Therapist:** If you find it particularly challenging to reduce digital usage, consider seeking help from a mental health professional.

Tip: Therapists can provide strategies to address underlying issues related to digital addiction, such as anxiety or depression.

- **Join Workshops or Seminars:** Participate in workshops focused on digital wellness and habit change to gain new tools and perspectives.

Resource: Look for local workshops on digital detox or online webinars hosted by wellness experts.

9. Utilize Technology Wisely

- **Use Apps to Support Your Detox:** Leverage apps designed to promote digital wellness, such as "Forest," "Freedom," or "StayFocusd."

Tip: Set daily usage limits for specific apps to prevent overuse.

- **Enable Focus Modes:** Use built-in device features that block distracting apps during designated times.

Example: Activate "Do Not Disturb" mode during work hours to maintain focus.

10. Maintain a Positive Outlook

- **Focus on Benefits:** Remind yourself of the positive changes you're experiencing, such as improved relationships, better sleep, and increased productivity.

Tip: Create a list of benefits you've noticed since starting your digital detox and refer to it when feeling discouraged.

- **Stay Motivated:** Continuously seek inspiration through books, podcasts, or motivational speakers who advocate for digital wellness.

Resource: Listen to podcasts like "The Digital Minimalists" or read articles from reputable sources on digital wellness.

Case Studies and Real-Life Examples

To illustrate the effectiveness of these strategies, consider the following case studies:

Case Study 1: Emma's Battle with Social Media Addiction

Emma, a 25-year-old marketing professional, found herself spending upwards of five hours daily on social media platforms. This excessive use led to decreased productivity, anxiety, and strained relationships. Determined to regain control, Emma implemented a digital detox plan that included setting daily time limits, turning off non-essential notifications, and engaging in offline hobbies like painting and hiking. Despite initial challenges and a few relapses, Emma's consistent efforts led to a significant reduction in screen time, improved mental health, and stronger personal connections.

"I realized that my constant scrolling was draining me more than it was fulfilling. Setting limits and finding joy in offline activities transformed my daily life." – **Emma**

Case Study 2: Tom's Struggle with Work-Related Screen Time

Tom, a 40-year-old software engineer, struggled to disconnect from work-related digital tasks, even during off-hours. This constant connectivity resulted in burnout and poor sleep quality. Tom decided to establish clear work boundaries by setting a strict end time for work-related activities and designating weekends as digital-free periods. He also sought support from his employer to implement flexible work hours. While Tom faced difficulties adjusting initially, the structured approach helped him reduce burnout symptoms, improve sleep, and enhance his overall well-being.

"Setting boundaries was challenging, but it was essential for my mental and physical health. Now, I feel more balanced and energized." – **Tom**

Case Study 3: Sarah's Emotional Dependency on Digital Devices

Sarah, a 30-year-old graphic designer, used her smartphone as a primary coping mechanism for stress and loneliness. This dependency led to compulsive checking and interrupted her daily routines. Sarah sought professional help and joined a support group focused on digital wellness. She incorporated mindfulness practices and physical activities into her daily life, which helped her manage emotions without relying on digital devices. Over time, Sarah developed healthier coping mechanisms, reduced her screen time, and experienced improved emotional stability.

"I realized I was using my phone to numb my feelings. Finding healthier ways to cope made a huge difference in my emotional well-being." – **Sarah**

Practical Exercises to Overcome Challenges

Incorporate these exercises into your daily routine to actively engage with the strategies discussed and reinforce your commitment to overcoming challenges.

1. Challenge Tracker

Purpose: Monitor your progress and identify patterns that lead to challenges or relapses.

How to Use:

- Create a table with columns for Date, Trigger, Action Taken, Outcome, and Reflection.
- Each day, note any challenges you faced, how you responded, and the result of your actions.

Example:

Date	Trigger	Action Taken	Outcome	Reflection
2024-05-01	Boredom after work	Went for a walk instead of scrolling	Felt refreshed and relaxed	Realized physical activity helps
2024-05-02	Stress at work	Practiced deep breathing	Reduced anxiety levels	Deep breathing effective

2. Relapse Prevention Worksheet

Purpose: Plan ahead for potential setbacks and outline steps to recover quickly.

Sections:

- **Identify Potential Triggers:** List situations or emotions that may lead to relapse.

- **Develop Coping Strategies:** For each trigger, outline specific actions to take instead of reverting to old habits.

- **Recovery Steps:** Define steps to take if a relapse occurs, such as contacting a support person or engaging in a mindfulness exercise.

Example:

Trigger	Coping Strategy	Recovery Steps
Feeling stressed	Practice 5-minute meditation	Take a short walk and breathe deeply
Boredom	Engage in a hobby like drawing	Call a friend or family member
Social pressure	Communicate boundaries clearly	Remind yourself of your goals

3. Self-Reflection Journal Prompts

Purpose: Encourage deeper understanding of your digital habits and motivations.

Prompts:

1. What emotions drive you to use digital devices excessively?

2. How does digital overuse affect your relationships and daily life?

3. What benefits have you experienced since reducing your digital usage?

4. What strategies have been most effective in overcoming challenges?

5. How can you reinforce your commitment to maintaining healthy digital habits?

4. Digital Detox Success Plan

Purpose: Create a personalized plan that outlines your goals, strategies, and support systems.

Sections:

- **Goals:** Define what you want to achieve with your digital detox.

- **Strategies:** List the specific strategies you will implement to reach your goals.

- **Support System:** Identify the people and resources that will support you.

- **Timeline:** Set a timeline for achieving your goals, including short-term and long-term milestones.

- **Evaluation:** Plan regular check-ins to assess your progress and make necessary adjustments.

Example:

Section	Details
Goals	Reduce social media usage to 1 hour/day
Strategies	Set daily time limits, turn off notifications, engage in offline hobbies
Support System	Accountability partner, join a digital detox group
Timeline	Achieve goal within 4 weeks, review monthly
Evaluation	Weekly progress reviews, adjust strategies as needed

Overcoming Challenges in Enhancing Real-Life Connections

Strengthening real-life connections can present several challenges, especially in a digital-centric society. Here are strategies to overcome common obstacles:

1. Time Constraints

- **Prioritize Relationships:** Recognize the importance of relationships and make them a priority in your schedule.

Tip: Treat social interactions with the same importance as work meetings by scheduling them in advance.

- **Efficient Time Management:** Use effective time management techniques to balance social interactions with other responsibilities.

Technique: Utilize time-blocking to allocate specific periods for work, social activities, and personal time.

2. Social Anxiety and Shyness

- **Gradual Exposure:** Slowly increase your participation in social settings to build confidence.

Example: Start by attending small gatherings before

progressing to larger social events.

- **Seek Support:** Consider seeking support from a therapist or joining a social skills group to overcome anxiety.

Resource: Look for local support groups or online communities that focus on overcoming social anxiety.

3. Maintaining Consistency

- **Set Reminders:** Use calendars or reminders to ensure you consistently engage in social activities.

Tip: Schedule regular meetups with friends and set reminders to attend them.

- **Accountability Partners:** Partner with a friend to hold each other accountable for maintaining social commitments.

Example: Agree to check in weekly about your social activities and encourage each other to stay consistent.

4. Balancing Digital and Real-Life Interactions

- **Digital Boundaries:** Establish clear boundaries for digital usage to prevent it from encroaching on real-life interactions.

Example: Implement a "no phones at the dinner table" rule to enhance family conversations.

- **Intentional Use:** Use digital tools intentionally to support, rather than replace, real-life connections.

Tip: Use messaging apps to coordinate in-person meetups instead of relying solely on digital communication for relationships.

Case Studies and Real-Life Examples

To illustrate the transformative power of enhancing real-life connections, consider the following case studies:

Case Study 1: Emily's Journey to Reconnect

Emily, a 28-year-old art teacher, found herself feeling isolated despite having numerous online friends. Realizing the superficiality of her digital interactions, she decided to prioritize real-life connections. Emily joined a local art class and started attending weekly meetups. Through these activities, she developed meaningful friendships, experienced increased happiness, and felt more connected to her community.

"I thought I was connected online, but nothing compared to the depth of real-life friendships. Joining local groups changed everything." – **Emily**

Case Study 2: Michael's Strengthened Family Bonds

Michael, a 45-year-old manager, noticed that his family's interactions were becoming increasingly dominated by digital devices. Determined to improve his family's relationships, he implemented a "no-device dinner" rule and organized monthly family outings. These changes led to deeper conversations, stronger emotional bonds, and a more harmonious family dynamic.

"Disconnecting from screens during dinner allowed us to reconnect and truly enjoy each other's company." – **Michael**

Case Study 3: Lisa's Path to Meaningful Social Interactions

Lisa, a 35-year-old nurse, felt overwhelmed by her busy schedule and struggled to maintain meaningful relationships. She decided to streamline her digital usage and focus on quality over quantity in her social interactions. Lisa started hosting monthly game nights with close friends and volunteered at a local community center. These efforts not only strengthened her existing relationships but also introduced her to new, supportive friends.

"Focusing on quality time with friends and engaging in community

activities enriched my social life beyond what online interactions ever could." – **Lisa**

Implementing Strategies to Overcome Challenges: Actionable Steps

To help you integrate the strategies discussed into your life, here are practical steps to follow:

1. Conduct a Relationship Assessment

- **Evaluate Relationship Quality:** Reflect on the quality and depth of your existing relationships.

Exercise: Complete the "Relationship Quality Assessment" worksheet (see Appendix B) to identify strengths and areas for improvement in your relationships.

- **Identify Gaps:** Determine which relationships need strengthening and which new connections you wish to cultivate.

Reflection Prompt: Which relationships feel fulfilling, and which ones feel superficial or neglected?

2. Set Clear Relationship Goals

- **Define Objectives:** Clearly outline what you want to achieve in your relationships, such as deepening existing connections or expanding your social circle.

Example Goal: "I want to develop deeper connections with three close friends by spending more quality time together."

- **Create a Plan:** Develop a step-by-step plan to reach these goals, including specific actions and timelines.

Plan Example: Schedule bi-weekly coffee dates with friends and plan monthly social activities.

3. Take Initiative in Social Settings

- **Initiate Conversations:** Don't wait for others to reach out—take the first step in starting conversations and making plans.

Tip: Reach out to a friend you haven't spoken to in a while and suggest meeting up for a coffee.

- **Be Open and Approachable:** Cultivate a friendly demeanor to make it easier for others to connect with you.

Technique: Practice open body language, such as maintaining eye contact and smiling, to appear more approachable.

4. Allocate Dedicated Time for Relationships

- **Schedule Social Time:** Block out specific times in your calendar dedicated to social interactions.

Example: Set aside Friday evenings for social activities with friends or family.

- **Be Present:** During social activities, focus on being fully present and engaged with others.

Tip: Put away your phone and minimize distractions to enhance the quality of your interactions.

5. Practice Active Listening and Empathy

- **Listen Fully:** Give your full attention to the speaker without interrupting or planning your response.

Exercise: During conversations, focus on understanding the other person's perspective without interjecting your own opinions immediately.

- **Show Understanding:** Acknowledge and validate others' feelings and perspectives to foster trust and intimacy.

Example: Use phrases like "I understand how you feel" or "That sounds really challenging."

6. Engage in Shared Experiences

- **Plan Activities:** Organize activities that you and others enjoy, creating opportunities for bonding and shared memories.

Example: Host a game night, go hiking together, or participate in a local workshop.

- **Collaborate on Projects:** Work together on projects or goals that require teamwork and cooperation.

Tip: Start a book club or a community service project to engage with others around a common interest.

7. Practice Gratitude in Relationships

- **Express Thanks:** Regularly thank people for their support, presence, and contributions to your life.

Example: Send a heartfelt message or give a small gift to show appreciation for a friend's support.

- **Acknowledge Milestones:** Celebrate important milestones and achievements with your loved ones to strengthen bonds.

Tip: Remember birthdays, anniversaries, and other significant events by planning a special celebration or sending a thoughtful note.

Overcoming Challenges in Enhancing Real-Life Connections

Enhancing real-life connections can present several challenges, especially in a digital-centric society. Here are strategies to overcome common obstacles:

1. Time Constraints

- **Prioritize Relationships:** Recognize the importance

of relationships and make them a priority in your schedule.

Tip: Treat social interactions with the same importance as work meetings by scheduling them in advance.

- **Efficient Time Management:** Use effective time management techniques to balance social interactions with other responsibilities.

Technique: Utilize time-blocking to allocate specific periods for work, social activities, and personal time.

2. Social Anxiety and Shyness

- **Gradual Exposure:** Slowly increase your participation in social settings to build confidence.

Example: Start by attending small gatherings before progressing to larger social events.

- **Seek Support:** Consider seeking support from a therapist or joining a social skills group to overcome anxiety.

Resource: Look for local support groups or online communities that focus on overcoming social anxiety.

3. Maintaining Consistency

- **Set Reminders:** Use calendars or reminders to ensure you consistently engage in social activities.

Tip: Schedule regular meetups with friends and set reminders to attend them.

- **Accountability Partners:** Partner with a friend to hold each other accountable for maintaining social commitments.

Example: Agree to check in weekly about your social activities and encourage each other to stay consistent.

4. Balancing Digital and Real-Life Interactions

- **Digital Boundaries:** Establish clear boundaries for digital usage to prevent it from encroaching on real-life interactions.

Example: Implement a "no phones at the dinner table" rule to enhance family conversations.

- **Intentional Use:** Use digital tools intentionally to support, rather than replace, real-life connections.

Tip: Use messaging apps to coordinate in-person meetups instead of relying solely on digital communication for relationships.

Case Studies and Real-Life Examples

To illustrate the transformative power of enhancing real-life connections, consider the following case studies:

Case Study 1: Emily's Journey to Reconnect

Emily, a 28-year-old art teacher, found herself feeling isolated despite having numerous online friends. Realizing the superficiality of her digital interactions, she decided to prioritize real-life connections. Emily joined a local art class and started attending weekly meetups. Through these activities, she developed meaningful friendships, experienced increased happiness, and felt more connected to her community.

"I thought I was connected online, but nothing compared to the depth of real-life friendships. Joining local groups changed everything." – **Emily**

Case Study 2: Michael's Strengthened Family Bonds

Michael, a 45-year-old manager, noticed that his family's interactions were becoming increasingly dominated by digital devices. Determined to improve his family's relationships, he implemented a "no-device dinner" rule and organized monthly family outings. These changes led to deeper conversations, stronger emotional bonds, and a more harmonious family dynamic.

"Disconnecting from screens during dinner allowed us to reconnect and truly enjoy each other's company." – **Michael**

Case Study 3: Lisa's Path to Meaningful Social Interactions

Lisa, a 35-year-old nurse, felt overwhelmed by her busy schedule and struggled to maintain meaningful relationships. She decided to streamline her digital usage and focus on quality over quantity in her social interactions. Lisa started hosting monthly game nights with close friends and volunteered at a local community center. These efforts not only strengthened her existing relationships but also introduced her to new, supportive friends.

"Focusing on quality time with friends and engaging in community activities enriched my social life beyond what online interactions ever could." – **Lisa**

Implementing Strategies to Overcome Challenges: Actionable Steps

To help you integrate the strategies discussed into your life, here are practical steps to follow:

1. Conduct a Self-Assessment

- **Evaluate Your Relationship Quality:** Reflect on the quality and depth of your existing relationships.

  Exercise: Complete the "Relationship Quality Assessment" worksheet (see Appendix B) to identify strengths and areas for improvement in your relationships.

- **Identify Areas for Improvement:** Determine which relationships need strengthening and which new connections you wish to cultivate.

Reflection Prompt: Which relationships feel fulfilling, and which ones feel superficial or neglected?

2. Set Clear Relationship Goals

- **Define Objectives:** Clearly outline what you want to achieve in your relationships, such as deepening existing connections or expanding your social circle.

Example Goal: "I want to develop deeper connections with three close friends by spending more quality time together."

- **Create a Plan:** Develop a step-by-step plan to reach these goals, including specific actions and timelines.

Plan Example: Schedule bi-weekly coffee dates with friends and plan monthly social activities.

3. Take Initiative in Social Settings

- **Initiate Conversations:** Don't wait for others to reach out—take the first step in starting conversations and making plans.

Tip: Reach out to a friend you haven't spoken to in a while and suggest meeting up for a coffee.

- **Be Open and Approachable:** Cultivate a friendly demeanor to make it easier for others to connect with you.

Technique: Practice open body language, such as maintaining eye contact and smiling, to appear more approachable.

4. Allocate Dedicated Time for Relationships

- **Schedule Social Time:** Block out specific times in your calendar dedicated to social interactions.

Example: Set aside Friday evenings for social activities

with friends or family.

- **Be Present:** During social activities, focus on being fully present and engaged with others.

Tip: Put away your phone and minimize distractions to enhance the quality of your interactions.

5. Practice Active Listening and Empathy

- **Listen Fully:** Give your full attention to the speaker without interrupting or planning your response.

Exercise: During conversations, focus on understanding the other person's perspective without interjecting your own opinions immediately.

- **Show Understanding:** Acknowledge and validate others' feelings and perspectives to foster trust and intimacy.

Example: Use phrases like "I understand how you feel" or "That sounds really challenging."

6. Engage in Shared Experiences

- **Plan Activities:** Organize activities that you and others enjoy, creating opportunities for bonding and shared memories.

Example: Host a game night, go hiking together, or participate in a local workshop.

- **Collaborate on Projects:** Work together on projects or goals that require teamwork and cooperation.

Tip: Start a book club or a community service project to engage with others around a common interest.

7. Practice Gratitude in Relationships

- **Express Thanks:** Regularly thank people for their support, presence, and contributions to your life.

Example: Send a heartfelt message or give a small gift to show appreciation for a friend's support.

- **Acknowledge Milestones:** Celebrate important milestones and achievements with your loved ones to strengthen bonds.

Tip: Remember birthdays, anniversaries, and other significant events by planning a special celebration or sending a thoughtful note.

Overcoming Challenges in Enhancing Real-Life Connections

Enhancing real-life connections can present several challenges, especially in a digital-centric society. Here are strategies to overcome common obstacles:

1. Time Constraints

- **Prioritize Relationships:** Recognize the importance of relationships and make them a priority in your schedule.

Tip: Treat social interactions with the same importance as work meetings by scheduling them in advance.

- **Efficient Time Management:** Use effective time management techniques to balance social interactions with other responsibilities.

Technique: Utilize time-blocking to allocate specific periods for work, social activities, and personal time.

2. Social Anxiety and Shyness

- **Gradual Exposure:** Slowly increase your participation in social settings to build confidence.

Example: Start by attending small gatherings before progressing to larger social events.

- **Seek Support:** Consider seeking support from a

therapist or joining a social skills group to overcome anxiety.

Resource: Look for local support groups or online communities that focus on overcoming social anxiety.

3. Maintaining Consistency

- **Set Reminders:** Use calendars or reminders to ensure you consistently engage in social activities.

Tip: Schedule regular meetups with friends and set reminders to attend them.

- **Accountability Partners:** Partner with a friend to hold each other accountable for maintaining social commitments.

Example: Agree to check in weekly about your social activities and encourage each other to stay consistent.

4. Balancing Digital and Real-Life Interactions

- **Digital Boundaries:** Establish clear boundaries for digital usage to prevent it from encroaching on real-life interactions.

Example: Implement a "no phones at the dinner table" rule to enhance family conversations.

- **Intentional Use:** Use digital tools intentionally to support, rather than replace, real-life connections.

Tip: Use messaging apps to coordinate in-person meetups instead of relying solely on digital communication for relationships.

Case Studies and Real-Life Examples

To illustrate the transformative power of enhancing real-life connections, consider the following case studies:

Case Study 1: Emily's Journey to Reconnect

Emily, a 28-year-old art teacher, found herself feeling isolated despite having numerous online friends. Realizing the superficiality of her digital interactions, she decided to prioritize real-life connections. Emily joined a local art class and started attending weekly meetups. Through these activities, she developed meaningful friendships, experienced increased happiness, and felt more connected to her community.

"I thought I was connected online, but nothing compared to the depth of real-life friendships. Joining local groups changed everything." – **Emily**

Case Study 2: Michael's Strengthened Family Bonds

Michael, a 45-year-old manager, noticed that his family's interactions were becoming increasingly dominated by digital devices. Determined to improve his family's relationships, he implemented a "no-device dinner" rule and organized monthly family outings. These changes led to deeper conversations, stronger emotional bonds, and a more harmonious family dynamic.

"Disconnecting from screens during dinner allowed us to reconnect and truly enjoy each other's company." – **Michael**

Case Study 3: Lisa's Path to Meaningful Social Interactions

Lisa, a 35-year-old nurse, felt overwhelmed by her busy schedule and struggled to maintain meaningful relationships. She decided to streamline her digital usage and focus on quality over quantity in her social interactions. Lisa started hosting monthly game nights with close friends and volunteered at a local community center. These efforts not only strengthened her existing relationships but also introduced her to new, supportive friends.

"Focusing on quality time with friends and engaging in community activities enriched my social life beyond what online interactions ever could." – **Lisa**

Implementing Strategies to Overcome Challenges: Actionable Steps

To help you integrate the strategies discussed into your life, here are practical steps to follow:

1. Conduct a Self-Assessment

- **Evaluate Your Relationship Quality:** Reflect on the quality and depth of your existing relationships.

Exercise: Complete the "Relationship Quality Assessment" worksheet (see Appendix B) to identify strengths and areas for improvement in your relationships.

- **Identify Areas for Improvement:** Determine which relationships need strengthening and which new connections you wish to cultivate.

Reflection Prompt: Which relationships feel fulfilling, and which ones feel superficial or neglected?

2. Set Clear Relationship Goals

- **Define Objectives:** Clearly outline what you want to achieve in your relationships, such as deepening existing connections or expanding your social circle.

Example Goal: "I want to develop deeper connections with three close friends by spending more quality time together."

- **Create a Plan:** Develop a step-by-step plan to reach these goals, including specific actions and timelines.

Plan Example: Schedule bi-weekly coffee dates with friends and plan monthly social activities.

3. Take Initiative in Social Settings

- **Initiate Conversations:** Don't wait for others

to reach out—take the first step in starting conversations and making plans.

Tip: Reach out to a friend you haven't spoken to in a while and suggest meeting up for a coffee.

- **Be Open and Approachable:** Cultivate a friendly demeanor to make it easier for others to connect with you.

Technique: Practice open body language, such as maintaining eye contact and smiling, to appear more approachable.

4. Allocate Dedicated Time for Relationships

- **Schedule Social Time:** Block out specific times in your calendar dedicated to social interactions.

Example: Set aside Friday evenings for social activities with friends or family.

- **Be Present:** During social activities, focus on being fully present and engaged with others.

Tip: Put away your phone and minimize distractions to enhance the quality of your interactions.

5. Practice Active Listening and Empathy

- **Listen Fully:** Give your full attention to the speaker without interrupting or planning your response.

Exercise: During conversations, focus on understanding the other person's perspective without interjecting your own opinions immediately.

- **Show Understanding:** Acknowledge and validate others' feelings and perspectives to foster trust and intimacy.

Example: Use phrases like "I understand how you feel" or "That sounds really challenging."

6. Engage in Shared Experiences

- **Plan Activities:** Organize activities that you and others enjoy, creating opportunities for bonding and shared memories.

Example: Host a game night, go hiking together, or participate in a local workshop.

- **Collaborate on Projects:** Work together on projects or goals that require teamwork and cooperation.

Tip: Start a book club or a community service project to engage with others around a common interest.

7. Practice Gratitude in Relationships

- **Express Thanks:** Regularly thank people for their support, presence, and contributions to your life.

Example: Send a heartfelt message or give a small gift to show appreciation for a friend's support.

- **Acknowledge Milestones:** Celebrate important milestones and achievements with your loved ones to strengthen bonds.

Tip: Remember birthdays, anniversaries, and other significant events by planning a special celebration or sending a thoughtful note.

Overcoming Challenges in Enhancing Real-Life Connections

Enhancing real-life connections can present several challenges, especially in a digital-centric society. Here are strategies to overcome common obstacles:

1. Time Constraints

- **Prioritize Relationships:** Recognize the importance of relationships and make them a priority in your schedule.

Tip: Treat social interactions with the same importance as work meetings by scheduling them in advance.

- **Efficient Time Management:** Use effective time management techniques to balance social interactions with other responsibilities.

Technique: Utilize time-blocking to allocate specific periods for work, social activities, and personal time.

2. Social Anxiety and Shyness

- **Gradual Exposure:** Slowly increase your participation in social settings to build confidence.

Example: Start by attending small gatherings before progressing to larger social events.

- **Seek Support:** Consider seeking support from a therapist or joining a social skills group to overcome anxiety.

Resource: Look for local support groups or online communities that focus on overcoming social anxiety.

3. Maintaining Consistency

- **Set Reminders:** Use calendars or reminders to ensure you consistently engage in social activities.

Tip: Schedule regular meetups with friends and set reminders to attend them.

- **Accountability Partners:** Partner with a friend to hold each other accountable for maintaining social commitments.

Example: Agree to check in weekly about your social activities and encourage each other to stay consistent.

4. Balancing Digital and Real-Life Interactions

- **Digital Boundaries:** Establish clear boundaries for

digital usage to prevent it from encroaching on real-life interactions.

Example: Implement a "no phones at the dinner table" rule to enhance family conversations.

- **Intentional Use:** Use digital tools intentionally to support, rather than replace, real-life connections.

Tip: Use messaging apps to coordinate in-person meetups instead of relying solely on digital communication for relationships.

Case Studies and Real-Life Examples

To illustrate the transformative power of enhancing real-life connections, consider the following case studies:

Case Study 1: Emily's Journey to Reconnect

Emily, a 28-year-old art teacher, found herself feeling isolated despite having numerous online friends. Realizing the superficiality of her digital interactions, she decided to prioritize real-life connections. Emily joined a local art class and started attending weekly meetups. Through these activities, she developed meaningful friendships, experienced increased happiness, and felt more connected to her community.

"I thought I was connected online, but nothing compared to the depth of real-life friendships. Joining local groups changed everything." – **Emily**

Case Study 2: Michael's Strengthened Family Bonds

Michael, a 45-year-old manager, noticed that his family's interactions were becoming increasingly dominated by digital devices. Determined to improve his family's relationships, he implemented a "no-device dinner" rule and organized monthly family outings. These changes led to deeper conversations, stronger emotional bonds, and a more harmonious family dynamic.

"Disconnecting from screens during dinner allowed us to reconnect and truly enjoy each other's company." – **Michael**

Case Study 3: Lisa's Path to Meaningful Social Interactions

Lisa, a 35-year-old nurse, felt overwhelmed by her busy schedule and struggled to maintain meaningful relationships. She decided to streamline her digital usage and focus on quality over quantity in her social interactions. Lisa started hosting monthly game nights with close friends and volunteered at a local community center. These efforts not only strengthened her existing relationships but also introduced her to new, supportive friends.

"Focusing on quality time with friends and engaging in community activities enriched my social life beyond what online interactions ever could." – **Lisa**

Implementing Strategies to Overcome Challenges: Actionable Steps

To help you integrate the strategies discussed into your life, here are practical steps to follow:

1. Conduct a Self-Assessment

- **Evaluate Your Relationship Quality:** Reflect on the quality and depth of your existing relationships.

  Exercise: Complete the "Relationship Quality Assessment" worksheet (see Appendix B) to identify strengths and areas for improvement in your relationships.

- **Identify Areas for Improvement:** Determine which relationships need strengthening and which new connections you wish to cultivate.

  Reflection Prompt: Which relationships feel fulfilling, and which ones feel superficial or neglected?

2. Set Clear Relationship Goals

- **Define Objectives:** Clearly outline what you want to achieve in your relationships, such as deepening existing connections or expanding your social circle.

Example Goal: "I want to develop deeper connections with three close friends by spending more quality time together."

- **Create a Plan:** Develop a step-by-step plan to reach these goals, including specific actions and timelines.

Plan Example: Schedule bi-weekly coffee dates with friends and plan monthly social activities.

3. Take Initiative in Social Settings

- **Initiate Conversations:** Don't wait for others to reach out—take the first step in starting conversations and making plans.

Tip: Reach out to a friend you haven't spoken to in a while and suggest meeting up for a coffee.

- **Be Open and Approachable:** Cultivate a friendly demeanor to make it easier for others to connect with you.

Technique: Practice open body language, such as maintaining eye contact and smiling, to appear more approachable.

4. Allocate Dedicated Time for Relationships

- **Schedule Social Time:** Block out specific times in your calendar dedicated to social interactions.

Example: Set aside Friday evenings for social activities with friends or family.

- **Be Present:** During social activities, focus on being

fully present and engaged with others.

Tip: Put away your phone and minimize distractions to enhance the quality of your interactions.

5. Practice Active Listening and Empathy

- **Listen Fully:** Give your full attention to the speaker without interrupting or planning your response.

Exercise: During conversations, focus on understanding the other person's perspective without interjecting your own opinions immediately.

- **Show Understanding:** Acknowledge and validate others' feelings and perspectives to foster trust and intimacy.

Example: Use phrases like "I understand how you feel" or "That sounds really challenging."

6. Engage in Shared Experiences

- **Plan Activities:** Organize activities that you and others enjoy, creating opportunities for bonding and shared memories.

Example: Host a game night, go hiking together, or participate in a local workshop.

- **Collaborate on Projects:** Work together on projects or goals that require teamwork and cooperation.

Tip: Start a book club or a community service project to engage with others around a common interest.

7. Practice Gratitude in Relationships

- **Express Thanks:** Regularly thank people for their support, presence, and contributions to your life.

Example: Send a heartfelt message or give a small gift to show appreciation for a friend's support.

- **Acknowledge Milestones:** Celebrate important milestones and achievements with your loved ones to strengthen bonds.

Tip: Remember birthdays, anniversaries, and other significant events by planning a special celebration or sending a thoughtful note.

Overcoming Challenges in Enhancing Real-Life Connections

Enhancing real-life connections can present several challenges, especially in a digital-centric society. Here are strategies to overcome common obstacles:

1. Time Constraints

- **Prioritize Relationships:** Recognize the importance of relationships and make them a priority in your schedule.

Tip: Treat social interactions with the same importance as work meetings by scheduling them in advance.

- **Efficient Time Management:** Use effective time management techniques to balance social interactions with other responsibilities.

Technique: Utilize time-blocking to allocate specific periods for work, social activities, and personal time.

2. Social Anxiety and Shyness

- **Gradual Exposure:** Slowly increase your participation in social settings to build confidence.

Example: Start by attending small gatherings before progressing to larger social events.

- **Seek Support:** Consider seeking support from a therapist or joining a social skills group to overcome anxiety.

Resource: Look for local support groups or online communities that focus on overcoming social anxiety.

3. Maintaining Consistency

- **Set Reminders:** Use calendars or reminders to ensure you consistently engage in social activities.

Tip: Schedule regular meetups with friends and set reminders to attend them.

- **Accountability Partners:** Partner with a friend to hold each other accountable for maintaining social commitments.

Example: Agree to check in weekly about your social activities and encourage each other to stay consistent.

4. Balancing Digital and Real-Life Interactions

- **Digital Boundaries:** Establish clear boundaries for digital usage to prevent it from encroaching on real-life interactions.

Example: Implement a "no phones at the dinner table" rule to enhance family conversations.

- **Intentional Use:** Use digital tools intentionally to support, rather than replace, real-life connections.

Tip: Use messaging apps to coordinate in-person meetups instead of relying solely on digital communication for relationships.

Case Studies and Real-Life Examples

To illustrate the transformative power of enhancing real-life connections, consider the following case studies:

Case Study 1: Emily's Journey to Reconnect

Emily, a 28-year-old art teacher, found herself feeling isolated despite having numerous online friends. Realizing the superficiality of her digital interactions, she decided to prioritize real-life connections. Emily joined a local art class and started attending weekly meetups. Through these activities, she developed meaningful friendships, experienced increased happiness, and felt more connected to her community.

"I thought I was connected online, but nothing compared to the depth of real-life friendships. Joining local groups changed everything." – **Emily**

Case Study 2: Michael's Strengthened Family Bonds

Michael, a 45-year-old manager, noticed that his family's interactions were becoming increasingly dominated by digital devices. Determined to improve his family's relationships, he implemented a "no-device dinner" rule and organized monthly family outings. These changes led to deeper conversations, stronger emotional bonds, and a more harmonious family dynamic.

"Disconnecting from screens during dinner allowed us to reconnect and truly enjoy each other's company." – **Michael**

Case Study 3: Lisa's Path to Meaningful Social Interactions

Lisa, a 35-year-old nurse, felt overwhelmed by her busy schedule and struggled to maintain meaningful relationships. She decided to streamline her digital usage and focus on quality over quantity in her social interactions. Lisa started hosting monthly game nights with close friends and volunteered at a local community center. These efforts not only strengthened her existing relationships but also introduced her to new, supportive friends.

"Focusing on quality time with friends and engaging in community activities enriched my social life beyond what online interactions ever could." – **Lisa**

Implementing Strategies to Overcome Challenges: Actionable Steps

To help you integrate the strategies discussed into your life, here are practical steps to follow:

1. Conduct a Self-Assessment

- **Evaluate Your Relationship Quality:** Reflect on the quality and depth of your existing relationships.

Exercise: Complete the "Relationship Quality Assessment" worksheet (see Appendix B) to identify strengths and areas for improvement in your relationships.

- **Identify Areas for Improvement:** Determine which relationships need strengthening and which new connections you wish to cultivate.

Reflection Prompt: Which relationships feel fulfilling, and which ones feel superficial or neglected?

2. Set Clear Relationship Goals

- **Define Objectives:** Clearly outline what you want to achieve in your relationships, such as deepening existing connections or expanding your social circle.

Example Goal: "I want to develop deeper connections with three close friends by spending more quality time together."

- **Create a Plan:** Develop a step-by-step plan to reach these goals, including specific actions and timelines.

Plan Example: Schedule bi-weekly coffee dates with friends and plan monthly social activities.

3. Take Initiative in Social Settings

- **Initiate Conversations:** Don't wait for others to reach out—take the first step in starting conversations and making plans.

Tip: Reach out to a friend you haven't spoken to in a while and suggest meeting up for a coffee.

- **Be Open and Approachable:** Cultivate a friendly demeanor to make it easier for others to connect with you.

Technique: Practice open body language, such as maintaining eye contact and smiling, to appear more approachable.

4. Allocate Dedicated Time for Relationships

- **Schedule Social Time:** Block out specific times in your calendar dedicated to social interactions.

Example: Set aside Friday evenings for social activities with friends or family.

- **Be Present:** During social activities, focus on being fully present and engaged with others.

Tip: Put away your phone and minimize distractions to enhance the quality of your interactions.

5. Practice Active Listening and Empathy

- **Listen Fully:** Give your full attention to the speaker without interrupting or planning your response.

Exercise: During conversations, focus on understanding the other person's perspective without interjecting your own opinions immediately.

- **Show Understanding:** Acknowledge and validate others' feelings and perspectives to foster trust and intimacy.

Example: Use phrases like "I understand how you feel" or "That sounds really challenging."

6. Engage in Shared Experiences

- **Plan Activities:** Organize activities that you and others enjoy, creating opportunities for bonding and shared memories.

Example: Host a game night, go hiking together, or participate in a local workshop.

- **Collaborate on Projects:** Work together on projects or goals that require teamwork and cooperation.

Tip: Start a book club or a community service project to engage with others around a common interest.

7. Practice Gratitude in Relationships

- **Express Thanks:** Regularly thank people for their support, presence, and contributions to your life.

Example: Send a heartfelt message or give a small gift to show appreciation for a friend's support.

- **Acknowledge Milestones:** Celebrate important milestones and achievements with your loved ones to strengthen bonds.

Tip: Remember birthdays, anniversaries, and other significant events by planning a special celebration or sending a thoughtful note.

Overcoming Challenges in Enhancing Real-Life Connections

Enhancing real-life connections can present several challenges, especially in a digital-centric society. Here are strategies to overcome common obstacles:

1. Time Constraints

- **Prioritize Relationships:** Recognize the importance of relationships and make them a priority in your schedule.

Tip: Treat social interactions with the same importance

as work meetings by scheduling them in advance.

- **Efficient Time Management:** Use effective time management techniques to balance social interactions with other responsibilities.

Technique: Utilize time-blocking to allocate specific periods for work, social activities, and personal time.

2. Social Anxiety and Shyness

- **Gradual Exposure:** Slowly increase your participation in social settings to build confidence.

Example: Start by attending small gatherings before progressing to larger social events.

- **Seek Support:** Consider seeking support from a therapist or joining a social skills group to overcome anxiety.

Resource: Look for local support groups or online communities that focus on overcoming social anxiety.

3. Maintaining Consistency

- **Set Reminders:** Use calendars or reminders to ensure you consistently engage in social activities.

Tip: Schedule regular meetups with friends and set reminders to attend them.

- **Accountability Partners:** Partner with a friend to hold each other accountable for maintaining social commitments.

Example: Agree to check in weekly about your social activities and encourage each other to stay consistent.

4. Balancing Digital and Real-Life Interactions

- **Digital Boundaries:** Establish clear boundaries for digital usage to prevent it from encroaching on real-life interactions.

Example: Implement a "no phones at the dinner table" rule to enhance family conversations.

- **Intentional Use:** Use digital tools intentionally to support, rather than replace, real-life connections.

Tip: Use messaging apps to coordinate in-person meetups instead of relying solely on digital communication for relationships.

Case Studies and Real-Life Examples

To illustrate the transformative power of enhancing real-life connections, consider the following case studies:

Case Study 1: Emily's Journey to Reconnect

Emily, a 28-year-old art teacher, found herself feeling isolated despite having numerous online friends. Realizing the superficiality of her digital interactions, she decided to prioritize real-life connections. Emily joined a local art class and started attending weekly meetups. Through these activities, she developed meaningful friendships, experienced increased happiness, and felt more connected to her community.

"I thought I was connected online, but nothing compared to the depth of real-life friendships. Joining local groups changed everything." – **Emily**

Case Study 2: Michael's Strengthened Family Bonds

Michael, a 45-year-old manager, noticed that his family's interactions were becoming increasingly dominated by digital devices. Determined to improve his family's relationships, he implemented a "no-device dinner" rule and organized monthly family outings. These changes led to deeper conversations, stronger emotional bonds, and a more harmonious family dynamic.

"Disconnecting from screens during dinner allowed us to reconnect

and truly enjoy each other's company." – **Michael**

Case Study 3: Lisa's Path to Meaningful Social Interactions

Lisa, a 35-year-old nurse, felt overwhelmed by her busy schedule and struggled to maintain meaningful relationships. She decided to streamline her digital usage and focus on quality over quantity in her social interactions. Lisa started hosting monthly game nights with close friends and volunteered at a local community center. These efforts not only strengthened her existing relationships but also introduced her to new, supportive friends.

"Focusing on quality time with friends and engaging in community activities enriched my social life beyond what online interactions ever could." – **Lisa**

Implementing Strategies to Overcome Challenges: Actionable Steps

To help you integrate the strategies discussed into your life, here are practical steps to follow:

1. Conduct a Self-Assessment

- **Evaluate Your Relationship Quality:** Reflect on the quality and depth of your existing relationships.

  Exercise: Complete the "Relationship Quality Assessment" worksheet (see Appendix B) to identify strengths and areas for improvement in your relationships.

- **Identify Areas for Improvement:** Determine which relationships need strengthening and which new connections you wish to cultivate.

  Reflection Prompt: Which relationships feel fulfilling, and which ones feel superficial or neglected?

2. Set Clear Relationship Goals

- **Define Objectives:** Clearly outline what you want to achieve in your relationships, such as deepening existing connections or expanding your social circle.

Example Goal: "I want to develop deeper connections with three close friends by spending more quality time together."

- **Create a Plan:** Develop a step-by-step plan to reach these goals, including specific actions and timelines.

Plan Example: Schedule bi-weekly coffee dates with friends and plan monthly social activities.

3. Take Initiative in Social Settings

- **Initiate Conversations:** Don't wait for others to reach out—take the first step in starting conversations and making plans.

Tip: Reach out to a friend you haven't spoken to in a while and suggest meeting up for a coffee.

- **Be Open and Approachable:** Cultivate a friendly

CHAPTER 9: OVERCOMING CHALLENGES AND RELAPSE

Embarking on a digital detox journey is a commendable step toward reclaiming your mind and body from the grips of digital overuse. However, like any significant lifestyle change, it comes with its own set of challenges and potential setbacks. This chapter delves into the common obstacles you might encounter during your digital detox, explores the reasons behind relapses, and provides effective strategies to overcome these hurdles. By understanding and addressing these challenges, you can maintain your commitment and achieve lasting success in your journey toward a balanced digital lifestyle.

Understanding the Nature of Challenges and Relapse

Change, especially when it involves altering deeply ingrained habits, is rarely smooth. Challenges and occasional setbacks are natural parts of the transformation process. Recognizing that these hurdles are temporary and manageable can empower you to navigate them with resilience and determination.

1. Common Challenges in Digital Detox

Several obstacles can impede your progress during a digital detox. Understanding these challenges can help you prepare and develop strategies to address them effectively.

- **Habitual Patterns:** Long-standing habits of checking devices frequently can be hard to break.

- **Social Pressure:** Friends, family, and colleagues may unintentionally encourage excessive digital use.

- **Work Demands:** Professional responsibilities often require constant connectivity, making it difficult to limit screen time.

- **Emotional Triggers:** Stress, boredom, or loneliness can drive you to seek comfort in digital interactions.

- **Accessibility and Convenience:** The omnipresence of digital devices makes it easy to revert to old habits, especially in environments where technology is readily available.

2. The Psychology Behind Relapse

Relapse is a common phenomenon in behavior change processes. Understanding the psychological factors that contribute to relapse can help you develop strategies to prevent it.

- **Cognitive Dissonance:** Holding conflicting thoughts about your digital habits can lead to inconsistency in your efforts.

- **Lack of Immediate Rewards:** The benefits of digital detox, such as improved well-being, are often long-term, making it challenging to stay motivated.

- **All-or-Nothing Thinking:** Believing that any lapse means total failure can discourage continued efforts after a minor setback.

- **Emotional Coping Mechanism:** Using digital devices to manage negative emotions can reinforce dependency, making relapse more likely during stressful times.

Strategies to Overcome Challenges and Prevent Relapse

Successfully navigating challenges and preventing relapse requires a proactive approach, self-compassion, and the implementation of effective strategies. Here are comprehensive techniques to help you stay on track.

1. Develop a Strong Mindset

Cultivating a resilient and positive mindset is crucial for overcoming challenges and avoiding relapse.

- **Embrace a Growth Mindset:** View challenges as opportunities for growth rather than insurmountable obstacles. This perspective fosters resilience and adaptability.

"Every setback is a setup for a comeback."

- **Stay Patient and Persistent:** Understand that change takes time. Celebrate small victories and remain committed, even when progress seems slow.

"Consistency is more important than perfection."

- **Practice Self-Compassion:** Be kind to yourself during setbacks. Acknowledge your efforts and treat yourself with the same understanding you would offer a friend.

"It's okay to stumble; what matters is that you continue moving forward."

2. Implement Practical Strategies

Adopting specific strategies can help you manage challenges and reduce the likelihood of relapse.

a. Set Clear Boundaries

Establishing clear boundaries around digital usage can create a structured environment conducive to your detox goals.

- **Designate Tech-Free Zones:** Create spaces in your home where digital devices are not allowed, such as the dining room or bedroom.

- **Define Tech-Free Times:** Allocate specific periods during the day when you disconnect from all digital devices, such as during meals or one hour before bedtime.

- **Use Physical Barriers:** Keep devices out of immediate reach to reduce the temptation to check them frequently.

b. Create a Supportive Environment

Surrounding yourself with a supportive network can provide encouragement and accountability.

- **Communicate Your Goals:** Share your detox plans with friends and family to gain their understanding and support.

- **Find an Accountability Partner:** Partner with someone who shares similar goals to monitor each other's progress and offer mutual support.

- **Join Support Groups:** Participate in online or local groups focused on digital detox and wellness to connect with like-minded individuals.

c. Develop Healthy Coping Mechanisms

Replacing digital interactions with healthier alternatives can help you manage emotional triggers without reverting to old habits.

- **Engage in Physical Activity:** Exercise releases endorphins, which can improve your mood and reduce the urge to seek digital comfort.

- **Practice Mindfulness and Meditation:** These practices enhance self-awareness and emotional regulation, helping you respond to stress more effectively.

- **Pursue Hobbies:** Investing time in activities you enjoy can provide fulfillment and reduce reliance on digital devices for entertainment.

d. Manage Work and Professional Responsibilities

Balancing digital detox with work demands is essential for sustained success.

- **Set Work Boundaries:** Define specific times for work-related digital usage and avoid extending it beyond those periods.

- **Utilize Productivity Tools:** Use tools like task managers and focus apps to enhance productivity without increasing digital consumption.

- **Communicate with Employers:** Inform your employer about your detox goals and negotiate flexible work arrangements if necessary.

3. Develop Relapse Prevention Plans

Even with the best strategies, relapse can occur. Having a plan in place can help you recover quickly and get back on track.

- **Identify Warning Signs:** Recognize the early signs of potential relapse, such as increased stress or frequent device checking.

- **Have a Recovery Plan:** Outline specific steps to take if you find yourself slipping back into old habits, such as taking a short break or reaching out to a support person.

- **Learn from Setbacks:** Analyze what led to the

relapse and adjust your strategies accordingly to prevent future occurrences.

4. Foster Long-Term Commitment

Maintaining a digital detox is an ongoing process that requires sustained commitment and adaptability.

- **Regularly Reevaluate Goals:** Periodically assess your detox goals to ensure they align with your evolving needs and circumstances.

- **Stay Informed:** Keep abreast of the latest research and strategies related to digital wellness to enhance your approach.

- **Celebrate Progress:** Acknowledge and celebrate your achievements, no matter how small, to reinforce your commitment and motivation.

Case Studies and Real-Life Examples

To illustrate the effectiveness of these strategies, consider the following case studies:

Case Study 1: Emma's Battle with Social Media Addiction

Emma, a 25-year-old marketing professional, found herself spending upwards of five hours daily on social media platforms. This excessive use led to decreased productivity, anxiety, and strained relationships. Determined to regain control, Emma implemented a digital detox plan that included setting daily time limits, turning off non-essential notifications, and engaging in offline hobbies like painting and hiking. Despite initial challenges and a few relapses, Emma's consistent efforts led to a significant reduction in screen time, improved mental health, and stronger personal connections.

Case Study 2: Tom's Struggle with Work-Related Screen Time

Tom, a 40-year-old software engineer, struggled to disconnect from work-related digital tasks, even during off-hours. This constant connectivity resulted in burnout and poor sleep quality. Tom decided to establish clear work boundaries by setting a strict end time for work-related activities and designating weekends as digital-free periods. He also sought support from his employer to implement flexible work hours. While Tom faced difficulties adjusting initially, the structured approach helped him reduce burnout symptoms, improve sleep, and enhance his overall well-being.

Case Study 3: Sarah's Emotional Dependency on Digital Devices

Sarah, a 30-year-old graphic designer, used her smartphone as a primary coping mechanism for stress and loneliness. This dependency led to compulsive checking and interrupted her daily routines. Sarah sought professional help and joined a support group focused on digital wellness. She incorporated mindfulness practices and physical activities into her daily life, which helped her manage emotions without relying on digital devices. Over time, Sarah developed healthier coping mechanisms, reduced her screen time, and experienced improved emotional stability.

Implementing Strategies to Overcome Challenges: Actionable Steps

To help you integrate the strategies discussed into your life, here are practical steps to follow:

1. Conduct a Self-Assessment

- **Evaluate Your Digital Habits:** Reflect on your current digital usage patterns, identifying areas of overuse and triggers that lead to excessive screen time.

- **Identify Personal Challenges:** Determine the specific challenges you face in your digital detox journey, such as habitual device checking or work-related digital demands.

2. Set Realistic and Flexible Goals

- **Define Clear Objectives:** Establish specific, measurable goals that address your unique challenges, such as reducing social media usage by one hour daily or implementing device-free zones in your home.

- **Allow Flexibility:** Recognize that setbacks are part of the process and adjust your goals as needed to accommodate your progress and changing circumstances.

3. Develop a Comprehensive Support System

- **Communicate with Loved Ones:** Share your detox goals with friends and family to gain their understanding and support.

- **Find an Accountability Partner:** Partner with someone who shares similar goals to monitor each other's progress and offer mutual encouragement.

- **Join Support Groups:** Engage with communities focused on digital detox to connect with like-minded individuals and gain additional support.

4. Create a Structured Plan

- **Establish Boundaries:** Define specific times and spaces where digital devices are limited or prohibited.

- **Implement Practical Strategies:** Use techniques such as setting screen time limits, turning off non-essential notifications, and replacing digital activities with offline alternatives.

- **Schedule Regular Check-Ins:** Set aside time each week to review your progress, identify challenges, and adjust your strategies accordingly.

5. Practice Mindfulness and Self-Compassion

- **Engage in Mindfulness Practices:** Incorporate activities like meditation, deep breathing, or yoga to enhance self-awareness and emotional regulation.

- **Be Kind to Yourself:** Acknowledge your efforts and treat yourself with understanding and compassion, especially during setbacks.

6. Monitor Your Progress

- **Track Your Screen Time:** Use built-in device trackers or third-party apps to monitor your digital usage and assess your progress toward your goals.

- **Reflect on Your Experiences:** Maintain a journal to document your journey, noting successes, challenges, and insights gained along the way.

7. Adapt and Evolve

- **Stay Flexible:** Be willing to adjust your strategies based on what works best for you and your evolving needs.

- **Seek Continuous Improvement:** Continuously explore new techniques and strategies to enhance your digital detox efforts and overall well-being.

8. Utilize Practical Tools

- **Apps and Technology:** Leverage apps designed to limit screen time, block distracting websites, and promote digital wellness.

- **Physical Tools:** Use planners, journals, or habit trackers to organize your goals and monitor your progress effectively.

9. Engage in Continuous Learning

- **Stay Informed:** Read books, attend workshops, or follow reputable sources on digital wellness and behavior change to deepen your understanding and refine your strategies.

- **Educate Others:** Share your knowledge and experiences with others to reinforce your commitment and inspire those around you.

10. Celebrate Your Achievements

- **Acknowledge Milestones:** Recognize and celebrate your progress, no matter how small, to maintain motivation and reinforce positive behavior.

- **Reward Yourself:** Treat yourself to non-digital rewards, such as a favorite meal, a new book, or a day out in nature, to celebrate your successes.

Overcoming Challenges in Boosting Well-Being

Enhancing overall well-being through digital detox can present several challenges. Here are strategies to overcome common obstacles:

1. Dealing with Resistance to Change

- **Understand the Benefits:** Remind yourself of the positive outcomes that boosting your well-being can bring to your life.

- **Start Small:** Begin with manageable changes to build confidence and momentum.

2. Maintaining Consistency

- **Set Reminders:** Use alarms or notifications to remind yourself to adhere to your well-being routines.

- **Create Habits:** Incorporate well-being activities into your daily routine until they become habitual.

3. Managing Time Effectively

- **Prioritize Tasks:** Focus on high-priority tasks that align with your well-being goals.

- **Use Time Management Tools:** Utilize planners, calendars, or apps to organize your schedule and allocate time for well-being activities.

4. Coping with Setbacks

- **Stay Resilient:** Accept that setbacks are part of the journey and use them as learning opportunities.

- **Seek Support:** Reach out to your support network for encouragement and assistance during challenging times.

5. Balancing Digital and Non-Digital Activities

- **Intentional Scheduling:** Allocate specific times for digital activities and ensure ample time for non-digital engagements.

- **Mindful Transitions:** Transition mindfully between digital and non-digital activities to maintain balance and focus.

The Synergy of Digital Detox and Overall Well-Being

Digital detox and overall well-being are intrinsically linked, with each enhancing the other in a synergistic manner. By reducing digital overuse, you create the necessary space and mental clarity to focus on activities and habits that promote holistic health. In turn, improved well-being reinforces your commitment to maintaining a balanced digital lifestyle, creating a positive feedback loop that sustains your progress.

Conclusion: Embracing a Life of Enhanced Well-Being

Boosting overall well-being through digital detox is a transformative endeavor that touches every aspect of your life.

By addressing mental, emotional, physical, and social health, you create a foundation for a fulfilling and balanced existence. The strategies and insights provided in this chapter empower you to take intentional steps toward enhancing your well-being, fostering a harmonious relationship with technology, and embracing a life rich in health, happiness, and personal growth.

As you continue your digital detox journey, remember that the pursuit of well-being is ongoing. Stay committed to your goals, remain adaptable to change, and continuously seek opportunities for personal development. By doing so, you not only reclaim your mind and body from digital overuse but also cultivate a life of sustained well-being and fulfillment.

CHAPTER 10: SUSTAINING YOUR DIGITAL DETOX JOURNEY

Congratulations! You've reached the final chapter of "Digital Detox: Reclaiming Your Mind and Body in a Hyper-Connected World." By now, you've gained valuable insights into assessing your digital habits, understanding the science behind digital detox, creating personalized plans, practicing mindfulness, improving sleep, enhancing real-life connections, boosting overall well-being, and overcoming challenges and relapses. This chapter focuses on sustaining your digital detox journey, ensuring that the positive changes you've implemented become long-term habits that contribute to a balanced and fulfilling life.

The Importance of Sustaining Your Digital Detox

Achieving a digital detox is a significant milestone, but maintaining the benefits requires ongoing effort and commitment. Sustaining your digital detox ensures that the improvements in your mental, emotional, and physical well-being are lasting. It involves integrating digital wellness into your daily routine, adapting to new challenges, and continuously refining your strategies to align with your evolving needs.

1. The Long-Term Benefits of Sustained Digital Detox

- **Consistent Mental Clarity:** Ongoing digital detox practices help maintain a clear and focused mind, enhancing your ability to think critically and creatively.

- **Enhanced Emotional Stability:** Sustained efforts contribute to emotional resilience, reducing susceptibility to stress and anxiety.

- **Improved Physical Health:** Long-term reduction in screen time promotes a more active lifestyle, better posture, and healthier sleep patterns.

- **Deepened Relationships:** Maintaining real-life connections fosters stronger, more meaningful relationships, providing a robust support system.

- **Increased Productivity and Creativity:** Continuous focus and reduced distractions lead to sustained productivity and innovative thinking.

2. Integrating Digital Wellness into Daily Life

Incorporating digital wellness into your daily routine ensures that your digital detox remains a natural and seamless part of your lifestyle.

a. Establish Routine Digital-Free Practices

- **Morning Rituals:** Start your day with activities that don't involve screens, such as stretching, meditation, or journaling.

- **Evening Wind-Down:** Develop a pre-sleep routine that excludes digital devices, allowing your mind and body to relax and prepare for restful sleep.

- **Scheduled Breaks:** Incorporate regular digital-free periods throughout your day to recharge and prevent digital fatigue.

b. Create a Balanced Digital Schedule

- **Prioritize Essential Use:** Focus on using digital devices for essential tasks like work, communication, and learning, while minimizing non-essential use.

- **Time Blocking:** Allocate specific time blocks for digital activities and non-digital pursuits, ensuring a balanced distribution of your time and attention.

c. Embrace Digital Mindfulness

- **Intentional Consumption:** Continue practicing mindful consumption by choosing digital content that adds value to your life and aligns with your goals.

- **Purposeful Engagement:** Engage with digital tools and platforms purposefully, avoiding passive browsing or mindless scrolling.

3. Adapting to New Challenges

Life is dynamic, and new challenges can arise that may test your commitment to digital detox. Adapting to these challenges ensures that you can maintain your progress despite changing circumstances.

a. Handling Technological Advancements

- **Stay Informed:** Keep up with new technologies and trends to understand their potential impact on your digital habits.

- **Evaluate Necessity:** Assess whether new technologies align with your digital wellness goals and integrate them mindfully if needed.

b. Managing Increased Digital Demands

- **Set Boundaries:** Clearly define work and personal boundaries to prevent digital overuse, especially when work demands fluctuate.

- **Use Productivity Tools:** Leverage productivity tools that support your digital detox, such as focus apps or digital well-being features on your devices.

c. Navigating Social and Professional Expectations

- **Communicate Clearly:** Inform friends, family, and colleagues about your digital detox goals to manage expectations and gain their support.

- **Seek Balance:** Strive to balance social and professional interactions with your digital wellness practices, ensuring that you remain connected without overindulging.

4. Continuous Self-Assessment and Reflection

Regular self-assessment and reflection help you stay aligned with your digital detox goals and make necessary adjustments to your strategies.

a. Regular Check-Ins

- **Weekly Reviews:** Set aside time each week to review your digital usage, assess your progress, and identify areas for improvement.

- **Monthly Evaluations:** Conduct more in-depth evaluations monthly to track long-term trends and make significant adjustments to your plan if needed.

b. Reflective Practices

- **Journaling:** Maintain a journal to document your experiences, challenges, and successes throughout your digital detox journey.

- **Mindfulness Meditation:** Use meditation sessions to reflect on your relationship with technology and reinforce your commitment to digital wellness.

c. Adjusting Goals as Needed

- **Reevaluate Goals:** Periodically revisit your goals to ensure they remain relevant and achievable as your circumstances evolve.

- **Set New Objectives:** As you achieve your initial goals, set new ones to continue your growth and deepen your digital wellness practices.

5. Building a Supportive Community

A supportive community can provide encouragement, accountability, and shared experiences that bolster your digital detox efforts.

a. Engage with Like-Minded Individuals

- **Join Communities:** Participate in online forums, local groups, or workshops focused on digital wellness and detox.

- **Share Experiences:** Exchange tips, challenges, and successes with others on a similar journey to gain insights and support.

b. Enlist Accountability Partners

- **Partner Up:** Find a friend or family member who shares your digital detox goals to monitor each other's progress and offer mutual support.

- **Regular Check-Ins:** Schedule regular meetings or conversations with your accountability partner to discuss your progress and address any challenges.

c. Seek Professional Support

- **Therapists and Coaches:** If needed, seek guidance

from mental health professionals or digital wellness coaches to address deeper issues related to digital dependency.

- **Workshops and Seminars:** Attend educational events that provide strategies and tools for maintaining digital wellness.

6. Embracing Lifelong Digital Wellness

Digital detox is not a one-time event but a lifelong commitment to maintaining a balanced and healthy relationship with technology.

a. Adopt a Digital Wellness Mindset

- **Mindful Integration:** Integrate digital wellness into your mindset, viewing it as an essential aspect of your overall health and well-being.

- **Continuous Learning:** Stay curious and open to learning new strategies and practices that enhance your digital wellness.

b. Celebrate Your Journey

- **Acknowledge Milestones:** Celebrate the milestones you've achieved in your digital detox journey to reinforce your commitment and motivate continued progress.

- **Reward Yourself:** Treat yourself to non-digital rewards, such as a favorite hobby, a day out in nature, or a wellness retreat, to celebrate your achievements.

c. Inspire Others

- **Share Your Story:** Share your digital detox experiences with others to inspire and encourage them to embark on their own journeys.

- **Lead by Example:** Demonstrate the benefits of

digital wellness through your actions, influencing those around you to prioritize their own well-being.

Case Studies and Real-Life Examples

To illustrate the effectiveness of sustaining your digital detox journey, consider the following case studies:

Case Study 1: Jennifer's Long-Term Commitment to Digital Wellness

Jennifer, a 35-year-old entrepreneur, implemented a digital detox plan to improve her mental clarity and work-life balance. After initially reducing her screen time by 40%, Jennifer continued to refine her habits by setting daily digital-free periods, engaging in regular physical activity, and nurturing real-life relationships. Over two years, Jennifer maintained her digital wellness practices, resulting in sustained mental clarity, enhanced creativity in her business, and deeper personal relationships. Jennifer's long-term commitment showcases how integrating digital wellness into daily life can lead to lasting positive outcomes.

Case Study 2: Michael's Adaptive Digital Detox Strategy

Michael, a 28-year-old software developer, faced increasing digital demands as his career progressed. To sustain his digital detox, Michael adapted his strategies by incorporating flexible work boundaries, utilizing productivity tools, and seeking support from his employer and peers. When faced with periods of high workload, Michael leaned on his support system and adjusted his digital boundaries to maintain balance. His ability to adapt ensured that he continued to benefit from his digital detox, avoiding burnout and maintaining a healthy work-life balance.

Case Study 3: Laura's Holistic Digital Wellness Journey

Laura, a 42-year-old healthcare professional, embraced a holistic approach to digital detox by integrating mindfulness, physical health, and social connections into her routine. She regularly attended mindfulness workshops, maintained a consistent exercise regimen, and participated in community events that fostered real-life connections. Laura's comprehensive approach to digital wellness allowed her to sustain her detox efforts, leading to improved mental health, physical vitality, and a strong sense of community belonging.

Implementing Strategies to Sustain Your Digital Detox: Actionable Steps

To help you integrate the strategies discussed into your life, here are practical steps to follow:

1. Develop a Comprehensive Sustainability Plan

- **Assess Your Progress:** Regularly evaluate your digital detox journey to identify what's working and what needs adjustment.

- **Set Long-Term Goals:** Establish ongoing goals that focus on maintaining and enhancing your digital wellness practices.

- **Create a Vision Board:** Visualize your digital wellness goals by creating a vision board that reminds you of your commitment and aspirations.

2. Incorporate Daily Digital Wellness Practices

- **Morning Rituals:** Begin your day with activities that promote well-being without screens, such as meditation, stretching, or enjoying a healthy breakfast.

- **Evening Wind-Down:** Develop a pre-sleep routine that excludes digital devices, allowing your mind and body to relax and prepare for restful sleep.

- **Scheduled Breaks:** Incorporate regular digital-free periods throughout your day to recharge and prevent digital fatigue.

3. Engage in Continuous Learning and Adaptation

- **Stay Informed:** Keep up with the latest research and strategies related to digital wellness to refine your approach.

- **Attend Workshops:** Participate in workshops or seminars that offer new techniques and insights into maintaining digital wellness.

- **Read Books and Articles:** Continuously educate yourself by reading books and articles on digital detox, mindfulness, and holistic health.

4. Foster a Supportive Community

- **Connect with Like-Minded Individuals:** Engage with communities focused on digital wellness to share experiences and gain support.

- **Join Accountability Groups:** Participate in accountability groups that monitor and encourage each other's digital detox efforts.

- **Share Your Journey:** Communicate your experiences and progress with friends and family to inspire and motivate others.

5. Practice Mindfulness and Self-Compassion

- **Daily Mindfulness:** Incorporate mindfulness practices into your routine to enhance self-awareness and emotional regulation.

- **Be Kind to Yourself:** Treat yourself with understanding and compassion, especially during challenging times or setbacks.

- **Celebrate Successes:** Acknowledge and celebrate your achievements to reinforce positive behavior and maintain motivation.

6. Utilize Practical Tools and Resources

- **Habit Tracking Apps:** Use apps like Habitica or StickK to track your progress and stay accountable to your digital wellness goals.

- **Journaling:** Maintain a journal to document your digital detox journey, noting successes, challenges, and insights gained.

- **Supportive Technology:** Leverage technology that supports your digital detox, such as focus apps, blue light filters, and productivity tools.

7. Balance Digital and Non-Digital Activities

- **Diversify Your Interests:** Engage in a variety of non-digital activities that enrich your life, such as hobbies, sports, or creative pursuits.

- **Prioritize Real-Life Interactions:** Continue to nurture and prioritize face-to-face relationships over digital communication.

- **Mindful Transitions:** Transition mindfully between digital and non-digital activities to maintain balance and focus.

8. Reflect and Adapt

- **Regular Reflection:** Set aside time each week or month to reflect on your digital detox journey, assessing what's working and what needs adjustment.

- **Adapt to Changes:** Be willing to modify your strategies based on your evolving needs and circumstances, ensuring that your digital wellness practices remain effective.

9. Embrace a Growth Mindset

- **Learn from Setbacks:** View setbacks as opportunities to learn and grow, rather than as failures.

- **Stay Curious:** Maintain a sense of curiosity and openness to new strategies and practices that enhance your digital wellness.

- **Continuous Improvement:** Strive for continuous improvement in your relationship with technology, seeking ways to optimize your digital habits.

10. Inspire and Lead by Example

- **Share Your Success:** Inspire others by sharing your digital detox journey and the positive changes it has brought to your life.

- **Encourage Others:** Support friends and family members who are embarking on their own digital detox journeys, offering encouragement and guidance.

- **Lead with Intent:** Demonstrate the benefits of digital wellness through your actions, influencing those around you to prioritize their own well-being.

Overcoming Challenges in Sustaining Your Digital Detox

Sustaining your digital detox journey can present several challenges. Here are strategies to overcome common obstacles:

1. Dealing with Resistance to Change

- **Understand the Benefits:** Continuously remind yourself of the positive outcomes that sustained digital detox brings to your life.

- **Start Small:** Implement small, manageable changes to build confidence and gradually incorporate more significant adjustments.

2. Maintaining Motivation

- **Set Short-Term Goals:** Break down long-term goals into short-term objectives to maintain motivation and track progress.

- **Celebrate Achievements:** Regularly acknowledge and celebrate your successes, no matter how small, to reinforce positive behavior.

3. Balancing Responsibilities

- **Effective Time Management:** Use time management techniques to balance personal well-being with professional and personal responsibilities.

- **Delegate Tasks:** Delegate or outsource tasks when possible to reduce stress and free up time for well-being activities.

4. Handling Setbacks

- **Stay Resilient:** Accept that setbacks are part of the journey and use them as learning opportunities.

- **Seek Support:** Reach out to your support network for encouragement and assistance during challenging times.

5. Avoiding Burnout

- **Pace Yourself:** Gradually implement well-being practices to prevent feeling overwhelmed.

- **Incorporate Rest Days:** Allow yourself regular rest days to recharge and maintain balance.

The Synergy of Digital Detox and Overall Well-Being

Digital detox and overall well-being are intrinsically linked, with each enhancing the other in a synergistic manner. By reducing digital overuse, you create the necessary space and mental clarity to focus on activities and habits that promote holistic health. In turn, improved well-being reinforces your commitment to maintaining a balanced digital lifestyle, creating a positive feedback loop that sustains your progress.

Conclusion: Embracing Resilience in Your Digital Detox Journey

Sustaining your digital detox journey is a testament to your commitment to a balanced and fulfilling life. By integrating digital wellness into your daily routine, adapting to new challenges, continuously assessing your progress, and fostering a supportive community, you ensure that the positive changes you've made are enduring. Remember that the pursuit of digital wellness is an ongoing process that evolves with your life's circumstances and growth.

As you move forward, embrace resilience and adaptability, knowing that each step you take towards maintaining your digital detox contributes to your overall well-being. Celebrate your journey, learn from your experiences, and continue to prioritize your health and happiness. By doing so, you not only reclaim your mind and body from digital overuse but also cultivate a life rich in well-being, purpose, and meaningful connections.

CONCLUSION: RECLAIMING YOUR LIFE

As you reach the end of "Digital Detox: Reclaiming Your Mind and Body in a Hyper-Connected World," it's essential to reflect on the transformative journey you've undertaken. This book has guided you through understanding the pervasive impact of digital overuse, exploring the science behind digital detox, and implementing practical strategies to restore balance in your life. Now, it's time to consolidate your learnings, celebrate your progress, and envision a future where you maintain a healthy, harmonious relationship with technology.

Reflecting on Your Digital Detox Journey

Embarking on a digital detox is more than just reducing screen time; it's a commitment to enhancing every facet of your well-being. Throughout the chapters, you've learned to:

- **Assess and Understand Your Digital Habits:** By tracking and analyzing your screen time, you gained insights into how digital overuse affects your life.

- **Create Personalized Detox Plans:** Developing tailored strategies ensured that your approach was sustainable and aligned with your unique needs.

- **Embrace Mindfulness and Digital Minimalism:** Cultivating awareness and intentionality in your digital interactions fostered a deeper sense of presence and purpose.

- **Improve Sleep and Enhance Real-Life Connections:** Reducing digital interference led to better sleep quality and stronger, more meaningful relationships.

- **Boost Overall Well-Being:** Addressing mental, emotional, physical, and social health dimensions resulted in a holistic improvement in your quality of life.

- **Overcome Challenges and Prevent Relapse:** Building resilience and implementing effective strategies helped you navigate setbacks and maintain your progress.

Celebrating Your Progress

Every step you've taken toward digital detox is a testament to your dedication to self-improvement and well-being. Celebrate the victories, no matter how small:

- **Reduced Screen Time:** Acknowledge the hours you've saved and the freedom that comes with less digital dependency.

- **Enhanced Focus and Productivity:** Recognize the increased efficiency and the quality of work you're now able to achieve.

- **Improved Sleep Quality:** Appreciate the restful

nights and the energy you gain each morning.

- **Strengthened Relationships:** Value the deeper connections and meaningful interactions you now enjoy with loved ones.

- **Greater Emotional Stability:** Embrace the balanced emotional state and resilience you've cultivated.

Envisioning a Balanced Future

Reclaiming your life from digital overuse is an ongoing journey. As you move forward, keep these guiding principles in mind:

1. Maintain Digital Boundaries

Continue to set and uphold clear boundaries for digital usage. Whether it's designating tech-free zones or adhering to a digital curfew, these boundaries help preserve the balance you've achieved.

2. Cultivate Mindfulness

Stay present in your interactions and activities. Mindfulness not only enhances your digital detox but also enriches your daily experiences, making each moment more meaningful.

3. Prioritize Well-Being

Keep prioritizing your mental, emotional, and physical health. Engage in regular self-care practices, pursue hobbies, and maintain an active lifestyle to sustain your overall well-being.

4. Foster Meaningful Connections

Continue to nurture your real-life relationships. Invest time and effort in building and maintaining strong bonds with family, friends, and your community.

5. Adapt and Evolve

Life is dynamic, and your digital wellness practices should adapt accordingly. Regularly assess your digital habits, set new goals, and be open to refining your strategies to align with your evolving needs.

Embracing Lifelong Digital Wellness

Digital detox is not a destination but a lifelong commitment to maintaining a healthy relationship with technology. By integrating digital wellness into your daily routine, you ensure that technology serves as a tool for enhancement rather than a source of distraction or stress.

1. Continuous Learning

Stay informed about the latest research and strategies related to digital wellness. Engage with resources that support your ongoing journey, such as books, workshops, and online communities.

2. Lead by Example

Inspire others by embodying the principles of digital wellness. Share your experiences, support those around you, and contribute to creating a culture that values balanced digital interactions.

3. Stay Connected with Your Purpose

Align your digital usage with your personal values and goals. Let your purpose guide your interactions with technology, ensuring that every digital engagement contributes to your overall well-being.

Final Thoughts: Reclaiming Your Life

Reclaiming your life from digital overuse is a profound and empowering journey. It's about taking control of your time, attention, and well-being in an increasingly digital world. By implementing the strategies and insights from this book, you've equipped yourself with the tools to navigate the digital landscape mindfully and intentionally.

Remember that every step you take toward digital detox is a step toward a more balanced, fulfilling, and vibrant life. Embrace the freedom that comes with reduced digital dependency, cherish the connections you've strengthened, and continue to prioritize your well-being. As you move forward, let the principles of digital detox guide you, ensuring that technology enhances rather than hinders your journey toward a healthier, happier you.

9 798344 007601